Battling Death:

A Different Life

Battling Death:
A Different Life

Marie Kirchner Stone

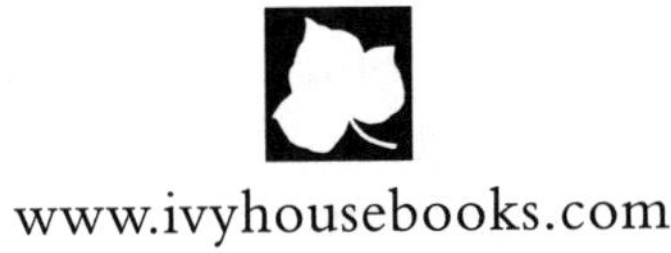

www.ivyhousebooks.com

PUBLISHED BY IVY HOUSE PUBLISHING GROUP
5122 Bur Oak Circle, Raleigh, NC 27612
United States of America
919-782-0281
www.ivyhousebooks.com

ISBN: 1-57197-422-9
Library of Congress Control Number: 2004103657

Printed in the United States of America

*To my parents,
my brother, Don, and
my sisters, Linda, LaVerne, Elvera, Donna, and Karen,
who always thought I didn't do enough.*

*To my colleagues,
who thought I did too much.*

*And to my students of 1966 to 1998,
whom I pushed to do more.*

Acknowledgement

Dr. Gordon Donn Mosser helped me intensively for five years during my first illness, in my early twenties. He also helped me as a friend for many years thereafter.

During the first series of treatments, Dr. Mosser met me in times as I battled Hodgkin's Disease. He also treated the internal and external problems caused by radiation. When the problems resulting mainly from radiation demanded oncological or gynecological referrals, Dr. Mosser made the recommendations.

Dr. Mosser and I began our physician-patient relationship with a dispute about my family's absence at early appointments, but Dr. Mosser gave in to my spunky remark, "I've been making my own decisions since I was fourteen, and I want to make these decisions on my own, too." That phrase pleased him and he often quoted it.

At age forty, Dr. Mosser was a teacher of resident radiologists and the author of articles on the treatment of Hodgkin's Disease. A well-known and respected clinician, he frequently argued with other senior radiologists about my treatment. At age eighty, he was still a snow skier and a fly fisherman. I appreciated what Dr. Mosser did for me, and he appreciated me because he was not only my physician, but also my friend, confidante, and adviser. It is to Dr. Mosser that I dedicate *Battling Death: A Different Life.*

Contents

Chapter Twelve, p.141
It Takes More than Ten Physicians to Heal a Patient

Chapter One

A Memoir Reflecting Fifty Years of Battling Illness

This memoir is the story of that sliver of my life that was dominated by my struggle with illness. I would not give in, so it is more a philosophy than a self-help book. My family taught me to preserve the privacy of others and my own privacy, which in the main I did; it was a principle I held sacred. It was my friends and colleagues who promoted my writing and broke my golden standard. My friends thought I had valuable information to share. I was hesitant to reveal facts about my own life and was often embarrassed to ask others impertinent questions. I was taught that each person owned his own narrative, which was his or her private business. Therefore, I did not include other patients.

In this memoir, I wish to explain how each decade, beginning when I was age 20 and lasting until age 60, surprised me with the attack of a new illness, which resulted in the loss of a favorite, important person, a husband, a lover, or a friend. I myself was surprised to contract illness after illness, decade after decade, but I counter-balanced illness with helping others through teaching. Teaching promoted a symbiotic, constructive, and mutually beneficial mind-body outcome both for the students and me.

My Fantasy—The Water Tower

The water tower was ironically the foundation of the lessons I learned. Teaching included Lesson One—teach courage; Lesson Two—to learn to battle the demons of illness through fantasy and imagination; Lesson Three—teach teacher and students to join in building self-esteem.

The grade school water tower was the embodiment of my imagination, especially when I ascended 150 feet into the air and stood at the top of it. I was usually dressed in blue jeans and a white cotton blouse, with my blonde braids flapping in the wind.

In the fifth grade, I was old enough not to endanger myself by climbing to the top of the water tower, but intellectually I had a vision of flying, motivated by the portrait of the angel that hung over my bed. I prayed to the angel nightly as a child; I had a hiatus from prayer, and returned again to pray as an adult. I didn't ask for anything, but communicated with the angel night after night using His prayer:

> Angel of God, my guardian dear,
> To whom His love commits me here.
> Ever this day be at my side
> To light and guard, to rule and guide.

Although not a Jewish prayer, this child-like prayer made me feel secure.

From the school water tower, the tower of my imagination, I observed the rooftops and still vividly envision that same fantasy fifty years later as I continue to battle with illness. My angel helped me to cultivate will, to triumph over adversity, the courage to prevail, and the imagination to invent stories. Any number of reasons made me want to climb the iron lattice steps attached to the six steel legs that held the water tower in position. When I reached the top of the tower, I fearfully stood up from my crouching position and felt the subtle sway of the tower under my legs.

Climbing the water tower caused my parents to punish me, and the school principal to threaten expulsion if I repeated acting like a stray cat that the firemen had to rescue. The truth was that I had climbed up and down the water tower when no one was watching. I thrived on these personal challenges no matter what my parents, the principal, or the firemen threatened. I taught students to trace the same challenges, emulating me. The water tower experiment helped me develop a backbone of inner steel in an experiment that didn't begin until age ten.

My first illness surprised me at age twenty. Imagination stabilized me through the different cancers and reproductive problems, open-heart surgery, pulmonary problems, and a body-consuming stroke. All illnesses continue to have residual effects today, five decades later.

Chapter Two

Teaching Becomes My Survival

The question was how to battle a different health problem each decade.

I said my childhood prayers nightly and clung to the prayers because they gave me a sense of stability even though I was not invested in god. My faith rested in children. Teaching became the source of my health, just like Lance Armstrong used "the bike as the thing," when he became ill with testicular cancer.

Teaching energized me after a bout with Hodgkin's Disease, a hysterectomy, thyroid cancer surgery, breast cancer, and gall bladder surgery. Teaching was my source of health for twenty-five years until I had open-heart surgery and a stroke. Then I was disqualified from teaching.

In Search of a Teaching Position

Late in the summer after college graduation, I seriously reflected upon teaching as a career. I began by searching for a position, but had difficulty securing one at such a late date in the summer. I finally found the perfect job; it was described in an advertisement in the *Minneapolis Tribune*. The advertisement read: "New High School Position Open! Experienced Teachers Only. Must Be Qualified to Collaborate with College Professors."

My meager teaching credentials and inexperience made me realize that I possessed inadequate qualifications for the position. In a quandary, I consulted the dean of my college, who also thought the position unattainable. Not easily deterred, and in spite of the dean's advice, I asked for and scheduled an interview. I ordered a taxicab to drive me to the new Alexander Ramsey High School in Roseville, a suburb of Minneapolis. The principal was unavailable because he was building the playground. He asked me to interview with the social studies' chairman, who was ordering maps. The superintendent was the only one available for an interview. I entered his office and the superintendent invited me to sit down on his new cream-colored leather sofa, that faced him.

Taking a deep breath, I tried to relax as Dr. Williams evaluated my credentials, which his secretary placed on the corner of his large, grey steel desk. He smiled and inquired, "Why teaching instead of women's retail?" The basis for the question was in my credentials, which acknowledged that I worked my way through high school and college selling women's clothing. I explained, "In women's retail, there seems to be less purpose. There is a dollar to be made, and it doesn't make much difference in the larger scheme of things whether the store across the street from our store profits or we do. By contrast, with teaching, what happens to just one student is significant."

The superintendent liked my answer, so he spent the next fifteen minutes sharing information about his new school.

The interview caused me to conclude that Alexander Ramsey High School was in a lower middle class suburb, comprised of families who were making their first debut toward the achievement of the American Dream. Their offspring were usually students from ethnic backgrounds.

These talented students often suffered from low self-esteem in contrast to their middle class partners, who were "born with silver spoons in their mouths." The new immigrants often squandered their intellectual gifts because their talents went unrecognized by teachers and parents alike. I made it my major goal to convert a student with a low self-esteem to one with a significant talent, focusing at times on playing a musical instrument, developing a science project, participating in athletics, or bilingualism. Superintendent Williams stated that most parents of children in the school completed high school only, and few completed college.

The superintendent closed my file and to my amazement, reached over the desk to shake my hand and offer me the position. He handed me a contract and a list of teachers' names with their phone numbers and addresses attached to enable me to contact the chairman of the social studies department, Jim Warren, so he could give me my teaching assignment.

Teaching was not my first love; it was women's fashion with which I became acquainted while working my way through high school. I was more the executive type with a knack for a "deal" than the professorial type with a scholarly manner. All aspects of women's fashion appealed to me. I liked clothes, had an eye for style, and appreciated aesthetics. The economics of fashion intrigued me as well as making a profit. The clerk had to be astute in knowing what and when to mark up or to mark down merchandise. I gained knowledge about the merchandise by closely observing when items emptied from the clothes racks. A retail position provided status in the community, especially when affiliated with style shows for which I wrote the scripts, selected the clothing, and chose the models.

By age sixteen, my salary averaged $20,000 annually, including commission. The salary increased incrementally. As I became an advanced salesperson, my commission increased exponentially. A salesperson's salary eclipsed a beginning teacher's salary tenfold. Retailing in a small women's store required a diverse set of skills and talents that teachers did not have or need. Besides selling merchandise, the skills included window decorating, advertising, marketing, tailoring, gift-wrapping, and all tasks to embellish the merchandise and its sale. I undertook many of these tasks to increase my salary. The goals between the two fields were diametrically opposed except for one pivotal element—both required selling, which was the art. From my viewpoint, the teacher's goal was to sell the children on the value of education; the retailer's goal was to sell the merchandise. My past experience demonstrated that too many teachers perpetrated a negative view rather than a positive influence on the pupils. Teachers often intimidated students without recognizing the pupils' needs.

For example, when I was a senior, I required a dictionary to complete my studies. When none were available in the classroom, I asked permission to go to the library to check out a dictionary. The teacher refused my request, informing me that I could use one from home. I couldn't understand her objection; we didn't have an extra dictionary at home that I could carry to school. I politely exited to the library in spite of her directive, but as I was leaving the room, the teacher spun me about and slapped me "smack" across the face. Horrified, I proceeded to the library, leaving the teacher to face her humiliation and the other students after she made a fool of herself. Such events increased my interest in education, which emerged slowly.

Ultimately, I attributed wanting to be a teacher to my mother, a volunteer teacher. On those days when she taught, she came home with a smile on her face. Mother taught elementary grades, but I preferred high school teaching. My objective was to convert mediocre achievers into excellent students. I also eventually wanted to become a college professor and teach teachers.

During my interview with Dr. Williams, I learned that the state of Minnesota required an annual medical check-up for new teachers. I had to postpone the physical evaluation because I obtained my teaching appointment too late in the fall to arrange for a timely medical appointment. Instead, I had to make the appointment during spring vacation, when I drove from Minneapolis home to St. Cloud to schedule a meeting with the family physician, Dr. Schwartz. I had a strange lump, the size of a small plum, at the base of the right side of my neck. But I was an optimistic person who had been healthy all my life. Before the doctor's appointment, I played a game of tennis with my former school friend at the city club to prove I was still healthy. Fortunately, I had my tennis clothes hanging in the car, making them available to play a game.

To impress my doctor, I dressed especially well to make him think I was healthy. The women's retail business taught me how clothes could masquerade appearances. I wore my white wool Easter suit, which I had been saving for an important occasion, and my natural straw hat covered with artificial red cherries. Sitting in the doctor's office, I nervously fiddled with the berries on my hat, which rested on my lap. I listened carefully to the physician's report, but heard only three words, "Hodgkin's Disease" and "cancer." I don't think I said anything, and I don't know what I felt. Hodgkin's Disease was unfamiliar, but sounded ominous, and the word *cancer* was both familiar and frightening.

In the 1950s, cancer evoked a similar emotional response as HIV does today in the twenty-first century. Although cancer was not contagious, people thought it was. True, death statistics were high and patients died from a variety of different cancers. Laymen wrongly, but fearfully, avoided the afflicted. For example, at lunch one day, my girlfriend wanted a sip of my Coke. She picked up my bottle from the table, but quickly returned it as fast with the apology, "I'm sorry but I don't want to catch cancer." Telling Dr. Schwartz about the incident at my next appointment, he advised me to anticipate more such responses—and he was right.

Dr. Schwartz, who had known me the first twenty years of my life, recommended that I see a radiation therapist because Hodgkin's Disease was not an internist's specialty. I requested the names of the three best radiation therapists at the University of Minnesota Hospital. I was yet too unsophisticated a consumer of medical care to ask for the names of the national authorities in the field of radiation therapy. I was also ignorant about the purpose served by a radiation therapist. The only physician I knew was the family internist. I accepted the list of names Dr. Schwartz provided, thanked him, and descended the office stairway. I'm unsure of the reason, but once outside, my bright sunny angel invigorated my spirit and energized my body. Out of nowhere, I seemed to have been propelled by a whirl of wind, which ignited my imagination. I added an extra lilt to my step and walked to the restaurant, deciding to eat lunch alone without my friend so I could recollect my thoughts in tranquility.

The habit of reflection always allowed me to invent various scenarios for action. For me, creative reflection was the first phase of problem solving, which I learned at age seventeen while working part-time in the Garment District of New York with a group of wise old Jewish retailers.

I arrived in the restaurant, sat at a luncheon table, ordered a glass of wine, and excavated my large Gucci bag in order to secure a sheet of paper from my notebook.

The second step in problem solving, that the same Jewish elders had taught me, was to make a task list to help gain control of a situation. I wrote, "Task one—learn about Hodgkin's disease; task two—select a good radiation therapist; task three—request a leave of absence from teaching; task four—break the rental lease on the apartment; task five—find a temporary residence near the University of Minnesota Hospital in order to live as an outpatient; task six—purchase a car . . . and the list went on. When I completed the list, I phoned my luncheon date to request a rain check and to suggest that we go for a ride later so that we could talk privately. He obliged.

Our mutual friends introduced us. My girlfriends were surprised that I finally began a relationship with a man whom I thought was "good enough for me." Unbeknownst to them, it was essential to me that his appearance was reminiscent of my grandfather, whom I idolized. Tim had been in the military during the Korean War before he entered the University of Minnesota, where he was now a student.

I believed him to be a man of character. He demonstrated intellectual curiosity, set high goals, and was a product of a well-bred family. He was the eldest of three children—having a younger brother and a younger sister.

He picked me up in front of the restaurant, gave me a modest hug, and drove off rapidly to park the car in a place where we could talk privately. He chose a parking place at the top of the hill overlooking the Mississippi River and the new bridge connecting the river's widest expanse between the east and the west. It was a breathtaking panoramic view. Looking down the embankment, I identified with the current that flowed steadily, dramatically, and powerfully southward. Nature was becoming my soul mate. With some difficulty, I formulated the words to tell my friend about my health problem. I was in denial, and repeating "Hodgkin's Disease" aloud made the illness more real. Most of my girlfriends spoke sweetly and expressed themselves in euphemisms. My truth, on the other hand, was called "brutal frankness." I didn't want the words "Hodgkin's Disease" to frighten and intimidate my friend, and I had no idea what his reaction might be. Finally, I turned to him and baldly announced, "I just returned from my annual checkup with Dr. Schwartz, who informed me that I have Hodgkin's Disease."

Five years my senior, world traveled, and sophisticated, my friend knew more about illnesses than did I. He asked about the evidence, and I reluctantly showed him the lump on my neck. He responded by reminding me, "You held high standards for others, and now we will hold you to those same high standards." I really did not know what he was talking about. What were the high standards I held for others? Who were the others? What did standards have to do with Hodgkin's Disease? Unsatisfied with our discussion, I politely asked him to drive me home, and on the way home, he reassured me of my strength, courage, and demonstrated capacity to manage problems. I refuted him because the other problems were of a different order of magnitude. In the long run, his answers were irrelevant because we stopped dating, and I learned that he, like most laymen, was uninformed and inexperienced about health problems. Both of us were in the childbearing years, and I wanted him to be free to fashion his life without me.

He returned to classes at the University of Minnesota, and his absence hurt me, but I approved.

When he abandoned me, his father befriended me. Some days I would be resting on the living room sofa in the late afternoons, and his father would deliver the evening newspaper. I was surprised and pleased by his father's gracious gesture to compensate for his son's leaving for Minneapolis so hastily.

Thereafter, I confined my male relationships to physicians, reasoning that physicians were knowledgeable about the causes and consequences of disease and required no special explanations. Unlike laymen, a physician could easily reject or accept me for my illness before a relationship broke my heart.

I spent several days in St. Cloud before returning to Minneapolis. Mother became curious because as yet she was uninformed about my diagnosis. I informed Mother that I had received critical news from the doctor, but added, "If you don't mind, I would like to explain the problem when I return home after visiting with my new radiologist." We did not have the conversation about Hodgkin's Disease that day or any other day. Without fanfare, I packed the two pieces of luggage, which I brought with me, placed them in my car, backed out from the driveway, and drove the ninety-minute return trip to Minneapolis to request a leave of absence from the superintendent of the Roseville School System.

Teaching in a Suburb (1956)

Sufficiently healthy to teach for several months, I continued in my position at Alexander Ramsey High School. The state of Minnesota was noted for its generally effective public school system, and the post-Sputnik era reinforced high educational standards.

The mid-1950s was a great time to begin a teaching career, and Alexander Ramsey High School was the place to commence teaching. The school was designed as one of the premier experimental institutions—a showcase school. The library was the central focus of the school, and research was the hub of intellectual activity. Students and teachers worked together in the library throughout the day, completing a newly developed research curriculum. The library provided classroom sets of books to facilitate an entire class. Students, therefore, had access to the total text for classroom study rather than a mere excerpt printed in a generic textbook. The textbook became obsolete at Alexander Ramsey High School.

Project-oriented study based on collaborative investigation dominated the curriculum. Teachers and students intellectually developed together. In one project, named Group Reading, the students from Grades 9-10 read selected texts chosen from science, social science, literature, and other humanities. Each class of twenty students dramatized their assigned text for the larger group of about one hundred students. The goal was to become acquainted with different genres on similar subjects. Students chose titles from among those presented by other students in the class. Many students enjoyed sharing their ideas with the members of the class and became avid readers of their favorite genres. Science fiction was just emerging as a new literature, and pupils were learning to appreciate it. In one demonstration class, a group of students clad itself in outer space clothing and built a robot to specification. The one hundred students were eager to enter the outer world atmosphere and to wear the clothing selected for them by the group in charge for the day. Some became astronauts or space men and others were robots walking on the moon. These space images pre-dated computer games. Little did students realize how closely the settings would soon simulate reality. Group Reading provided an introduction to immersion learning, which today continues at a number of universities from Colorado College to Harvard University.

The teachers at Alexander Ramsey were chosen for their talent, credentials, and experience. Some became

University of Minnesota professors who team-taught university undergraduates while teaching new teachers in training for Alexander Ramsey High School. The young teachers, assisted by mature master teachers, developed effective styles and methods of interdisciplinary curriculum. University teaching became very satisfying to me.

Principal Curtis Johnson, a renowned educator, initiated another new type of program. At mid-day, all three levels of students participated in an activity of their choice selected from among some thirty or more courses. I enjoyed teaching this experimental block the most and learned from the approach how to combine national and world events, literature and history, and the arts and other humanities. For the mid-day session, I created a course called LIDRAMUSARTS, standing for the combination of literature, drama, music, and art, designed for students interested in or majoring in the arts. A group of students in the class assisted in developing the course. We selected, interviewed, and invited guests for a scheduled monthly two-hour session to lecture and perform. The number in class grew larger by the week, and some of our guest speakers presented evening performances. We were fortunate to draw from the University of Minnesota, the new Guthrie Theater, the Minneapolis Symphony, the Walker Art Center, and other cultural institutions in the Alexander Ramsey High School's backyard. Sir Tyrone Guthrie, Jessica Tandy, George Grizzard, Alonzo Hauser, Frederick Fennel, and other luminaries accepted our invitations to perform. The Walker Art Center presented demonstration classes with live models for young sculptors. Teaching at an experimental school was exhilarating and acquainted me with new approaches to teaching and learning.

It was the psychology department that taught me the value of familiarizing myself with the strengths and weaknesses of each student. At the beginning of each term, I was taught to review the personnel folders of all students in my courses and to identify, in summary form on a three-by-five card, significant points to remember about each student. The high caliber of the teaching staff demonstrated that teachers could accomplish great feats with students. My commitment to teaching doubled.

Teachers often talked in the lunchroom over the lunch hour. Sometimes after school, a half dozen teachers would go for a glass of wine to talk about teaching until it became dark outside. My socializing was usually affiliated with teaching.

Each day, I liked teaching more and more and regretted leaving the retail business less and less. Now, because of Hodgkin's Disease, I had to leave classroom teaching after only several months of experience, but I requested, and was granted, a leave of absence by Superintendent Williams with his caveat, "You may return to teach when you again are healthy because you are a natural born teacher." I was flattered.

After ending my contract with Alexander Ramsey High School, I exited the school and entered my newly purchased convertible, and drove to my apartment on the south side of Minneapolis to cancel the lease I made that fall with two new roommates who had recently moved to Minneapolis from Canada. I didn't yet know my new roommates very well, so it was mainly a financial transaction rather than a personal one.

Both roommates were shocked by my diagnosis and found it hard to accept. I left the apartment in tears—theirs and mine—got into my car, and drove north across town to the university campus where I parked my car in the hospital parking lot. I was twenty minutes early for my three o'clock doctor's appointment. Waiting, I sat in my car, highly disturbed and agitated by the anguishing sensation that I had successfully invented a life during the past half year and now I had to close it out. I wasted six months getting my life and career in shape, but my success was in vain. I lost health, I lost my new teaching position, I lost my apartment, and I lost the man I liked. I was told that I had Hodgkin's Disease, but that was the only evidence I had of being sick. I certainly did not feel different from the days when I was well. I didn't feel or look any different from the healthy teachers, who were shocked to hear the news that I was leaving my position because of cancer. I dressed particularly well the day I announced my illness to the faculty. I had to begin another life with little knowledge about the nature of my undertaking.

The one thing I learned was that teaching could become my survival. Each time I became well enough to teach, I sought a new teaching position. My goal was to create a purposeful life through teaching children. I taught in a variety of positions—one public school, two private schools, and two universities throughout five decades of teaching.

Hodgkin's Disease Lays a Different Foundation (Early 1958)

With trepidation, I locked the car and descended the stairs to the sub-basement of the University of Minnesota

Hospital, where I first met Dr. Mosser in the office of the Radiology Department. Dr. Mosser realized it was my first visit, and to impress him, I dressed in a navy sailor sweater and jacket with a matching short, tight white skirt. Dr. Mosser shook my hand cordially, introduced himself, and looking about asked, "Are your parents still parking the car?" I replied, "No, they won't be joining us." I added, "I want to decide on the treatment myself. I've made all my own decisions since I was fourteen and want to make these decisions, too." With a shocked look, Dr. Mosser responded, "You're a brave young lady, but life and death decisions are of a different level of magnitude from the decisions you're used to making. Do you know what Hodgkin's Disease is? What radiation treatments are? What their results can be?" I answered, "No, but I guess you will tell me." Walking behind his desk, he placed his horn rim glasses on the top of his balding head and in a serious and hesitant tone, he informed me, "Some patients live several months from the onset of this illness, the majority of patients die within two to five years, and a small percentage lives between ten and twenty years." I quipped, "I've always been an outlier, so chances are that I will die in the first months or live for ten years." It was bravado talking, but I wanted to convince Dr. Mosser that I relied on his professional judgment and my own, not on my family's judgment. I neglected to explain to him that as of yet, I had avoided informing my family about the diagnosis of cancer. After some dispute, Dr. Mosser conceded that it wasn't essential that my parents attend the first meeting. He continued by explaining the nature of Hodgkin's Disease in layman's terms, presenting me with a duplicate two-page description from a medical text on Hodgkin's Disease to read and share with my parents.

Description of Hodgkin's Disease

Hodgkin's Disease is a relatively uncommon malignant lymphoma. The disease is a chronic disorder of unknown etiology, involving the lymphatic and immune systems. Common to both are lymphocytes, which are the immune cells that are abnormal in the Hodgkin's patient.

Thousands of lymph nodes are connected to a lymphatic drainage system that facilitates removal from the body of particulate matter derived from injuries, infections, and normal cell turnover. The affliction of this system is the essence of Hodgkin's Disease. The disorder affects children, adolescents, males, females, and adults of all ages.

Its clinical presentation includes fever and enlargement of the lymph nodes and spleen. While Hodgkin's Disease is generally classified as a malignant lymphoma, it is not a cancer in the conventional sense because the lymphocytes do not show the microscopic presence of mitosis, dedifferentiation, and invasiveness usual in cancer. Nevertheless, if untreated, it shares with cancer a malignant course.

In 1932, Thomas Hodgkin originally described the disease, and radiation was the sole treatment. In the 1930s, some radiotherapists began to effectively use high doses of radiation over greater areas of the body. In 1956, Dr. Henry Kaplan at Stanford University acquired the first medical linear accelerator in the western hemisphere, which allowed delivery of mega doses of radiation to deep tissues while limiting radiation injury to the skin. Treatment for Hodgkin's Disease advanced significantly beginning in the 1960s as physicians recognized the need to determine the extent of the disease according to the organs affected and the number and location the chains of lymph nodes involved. This staging of the disease predicts its outcome and dictates the type and duration of treatment.

Four stages of disease severity were identified. Stage I disease is limited to a single chain of lymph nodes usually in the neck or axilla. Stage II disease involves two or more lymph node collections above the diaphragm. These two stages are treated by radiating the neck, scapula, mediastinum, and underarms in a shawl-like style. Stage III disease involves nodes above and beneath the diaphragm, which is treated in a Y-shape. Stage IV disease afflicts body organs such as the lungs, liver, and spleen, as well as the lymph nodes. The most serious form of Hodgkin's Disease is treated by total nodal irradiation.

In the early 1970s, newly developed chemo-therapeutic drugs, alone or in combination with radiation, became the accepted mode of treatment, and in 1971, the use of a CT (Computerized Axial Tomography) scan gave a more sensitive and quantitative imaging technique for staging.

Prior to the 1960s, death from Hodgkin's Disease followed a typical bell shape distribution. Most patients died within two to five years of diagnosis. The remainder succumbed within weeks to months following an especially virulent course, while a small group lived sometimes ten to twenty years.

Current chemotherapy and radiation therapy has vastly improved the outcome. Cure rates of ninety percent are now achievable, but the final outcome is often dictated by the long term consequences of the treatment. The dramatic improvement in outcomes is tempered by the complications of treatment.

Irradiated patients are at risk for secondary malignancies like melanoma, breast, lung, and thyroid
cancer. Because radiation injures normal tissue, it can
give rise to serious heart and lung problems or skin
cancers."[1]

From my perspective, the textbook description of
Hodgkin's was painted with a dark brush, but I still found
a hopeful message. Unfortunately, I was diagnosed with
Hodgkin's Disease several years before advancements in
the field were made. The timing for illness is never good,
but this was a particularly deleterious time. I just missed
the breakthrough in treatment that began in 1956 with the
linear accelerator.

Therapy for Hodgkin's Disease (1958–1961)

My treatment was limited exclusively to radiotherapy
because at that time, the University of Minnesota had no
linear accelerator and was not yet using chemotherapy. The
treatment was based on the delivery of roentgens, now
called rads, applied by a Picker Cobalt machine.

At the onset of the treatments, Dr. Mosser helped me
find an apartment in a sorority house within walking distance from the hospital to enable me to be an outpatient.
He had many connections and offered his help effortlessly.

---

[1] This description was gleaned from a lengthy conversation the author
had with an internist-hematologist knowledgeable about the disease.
Additional information about Hodgkin's disease can be found in the
Merck Manual of Medical Information, Robert Berkow, Mark H. Beers, and
Andrew J. Fletcher, Eds. Pocket Books, New York, 1997, pp. 846–849.

I suffered from Stage II Hodgkin's Disease, and on the first day I arrived for treatment, Dr. Mosser informed me that he, with the assistance of a resident, would radiate me in a shawl-like profile to enable radiation of my neck, chest, back, and under arms. When I entered the small, enclosed radiation room, the resident asked that I change into a hospital gown and lie on the table quietly. When prone, the resident measured the areas he wanted to treat and covered the remainder of my body with heavy lead pads made of a gray rubber-like substance to block the radiation from the healthy parts of my body. I had to lay very still because if I moved, the resident, who peered through a two-foot square window, stopped the cobalt machine and ended the treatment. "The treatment process," the resident explained, "hurts less than a slap across the buttocks." In fact, the treatment per se did not hurt at all; it was the results of the treatments that caused pain. Radiation treatments lasted for only fifteen or twenty minutes each. I spent the remainder of most days sleeping or reading, having little energy to do much else.

The treatments nauseated me, and each day resulted in greater physical discomfort. As the weeks passed, my entire body writhed in pain. The cobalt machine caused severe radiation burns as the rads melted the cancerous Hodgkin's chains. It seemed cruel to radiate me day after day until I was like a crisp oven-roasted bird.

My instinct was to revolt and stop the treatments because they were intolerable. I had to persuade myself to continue. I used a little technique to alleviate some pain. I counted the number of treatments backwards instead of forwards to pretend that I had fewer to complete. Upon completion of a session, for instance, I would calculate "another twenty minutes," "another day," "another week," rather than counting forward—twenty more weeks to go, ten more weeks to go, or the number of treatments yet to endure. Little tricks helped a little bit.

Nothing occupied the twenty-minute radiation therapy session except staring at the four gray walls. The treatment cubicle was painted a dark depressing gray, and I recommended that the hospital janitors paint the walls yellow to add cheer. During my years of treatment, the walls remained gray; the patients' wishes were disregarded in those days. Later I tried anew, requesting that the hospital staff play music, audible in the cubicle—Mozart, Chopin, Ravel—but Dr. Mosser informed me that a radio had been tried, and it became a nuisance because patients argued about what genre of music to play. I was told changing stations frequently distracted and wasted the residents' time. Not easily defeated, I invented several of my own games. One invention used numbers, such as naming ten books in numerical order—*One Enchanted Evening, Two Faces of Eve, Three Days in May, Four Horsemen of the Apocalypse*, etc. Another game used the alphabet, asking the player to list twenty philosophers in alphabetic order. Still, a third game used history and requested names of famous people who lived in a given historical period, like ten biographies about leaders in World War II. I planned to maintain the game formats and publish a book that would be titled *What to Do Instead of Counting Sheep*. The mind games occupied radiation periods and eliminated boredom temporarily.

Being daily shut in a room that measured less than ten feet long caused a mild case of claustrophobia that spilled into other small spaces like bathrooms, elevators, airplanes, and sometimes even crowded larger spaces. Eventually, I overcame a degree of claustrophobia, but today I still suffer a lingering hangover, which at times causes me to panic. For instance, I insist on open doors at all times.

Five months of treatments five days a week between August and Christmas 1958 resulted in visible scarring. I don't know what came first, the skin burns, the weight loss and frequent regurgitation, the loss of my thick sandy blonde hair, or coughing. A single problem was anguishing, but the attack of multiple problems in an unpredictable sequence caused great physical and emotional devastation. I felt as if God transformed the biblical plagues, cast them in contemporary settings, and applied them to test me. For each plague, I created an aesthetic solution, the same way I tried to fool the doctors by overdressing for appointments. I was vain about my appearance and searched for creative cover-ups that made me feel better.

The first plague was weight loss. Thin already, this plague caused me to lose forty pounds and only my Bermuda shorts and blazers were bulky enough to camouflage my weight loss. To compensate for the weight loss I ate small portions of food frequently and with great dedication. I returned to 110 pounds. Thin was appealing to me, so I tried to create a look for "You can't be too rich or too thin," which was a cigarette advertisement from that era. My signature garment was a wardrobe of gathered cotton gauze skirts with matching gauze jackets; Bermuda shorts with blazers; or T-shirts and tight fitting sleek slacks.

The second "plague" was skin burns. The radiated parts of my body began to change from a bright pink to a deep purple as the depth of the burn increased. I knew the burns would worsen with each treatment and eventually become dead tissue that had to be debrided. I learned to wear men's white cotton shirts, which provided a loose cover to protect against infection. I combined the white shirts with different color small cotton scarves I tied around my purple neck to hide it. Women wearing men's shirts was not the fashion of the fifties, but I had a flair for making things fashionable. Soon, healthy girls imitated me by wearing men's white shirts with cotton scarves. It was flattering to be imitated, and after awhile, the girls did not bother to inquire about the cause of the deep purple scars on my neck, but asked about where to purchase the shirts and scarves.

God hoisted the third "plague" on me by causing me to lose my hair. In the beginning, small bunches of hair came out in my comb. Then one day to my utter dismay, I stared in the mirror and pulled out thick handfuls of sandy blonde hair. My choices were to scream or to cry and I did both because I was very angry. My sexuality was integrally related to my hair, and I desperately needed to solve the problem. Without hair, I felt masculine. I had a theory, "You didn't need to be good looking, but you had to develop a good look," which I tried to create. The cropped hairstyle of the 2000s was not yet fashionable.

Finally admitting I would be bald, I investigated solutions from beauticians, physicians, professionals, and other patients, but these usual sources knew little about hair replacement in the 1950s, even if hair replacement was essential to their professional services. I called the American Cancer Society, requesting its catalog, but I disliked the "old lady" wigs they featured. I had little money, but I commissioned expensive, natural hair wigs and falls, which I ordered from Darcel's, a New York salon where I met the famous songstress, Lena Horne. My thinking was, "If Darcel's Salon is good enough for Lena Horne, it has to be good enough for me." Beautiful and successful, Lena Horne, the first woman I met who wore wigs, offered encouragement when we chatted over cups of coffee on my trips to New York that coincided with her appointments at Darcel's. I finally decided the cost of purchase and care for natural hairpieces was prohibitive for me, so I experimented with artificial wigs at about a third of the cost. The problem with artificial wigs was they required frequent washing and setting and had to be washed at the beauty salon. I finally solved the hair problem by purchasing seven inexpensive artificial wigs, which I placed on wig stands on the closet shelf and alternated wearing and cleaning them every three days. Without knowledge, experience, or someone familiar with the problem, trial and error was the only teacher for the purchase of wigs and the solution to other problems. Some days I had to ask my dear, dear friend, Sue Ettelson, to help me. She always found new wigs and had the soiled wigs shampooed.

After several years, I no longer had a need for wigs because the remains of my straight, sandy blonde hair disappeared and nature replaced it with thick, dark brunette curly hair. I lost my hair several times thereafter, but it always returned thick, brunette, and curly. Ironically, when my natural hair grew back, my friends mistook the natural hair for a wig. In fact, I comfortably learned to wear wigs and did so at certain times thereafter for reasons of vanity. Artificial wigs presented the best solution for hairpieces, but I did not solve the sexuality issue caused by the absence of hair.

The worst "plague" imposed was coughing. I had always enjoyed a big booming voice that I could project across the auditorium when I was teaching. Now I coughed until I thought I would choke. Coughing took great energy and could not be suppressed. Medications did not help. Eventually, I lost my voice, but I did regain it.

Hairless, voiceless, and skinny was a difficult triumvirate to battle. The skin burns encircled my neck, voice problems plagued my throat, and I soon forgot how I initially looked. The worst problem was my loss of sexual identity caused by loss of hair, which made me feel utterly masculine. I adapted to each problem, spending years struggling with my appearance and trying to make myself well by looking good. The appearance problems consumed more time than the physical problems, but the distinction is actually irrelevant because one was the manifestation of the other. I became my own shadow—my ghost—questioning if I was Job challenged by plagues or Lazarus raised from the dead. Often I referred to myself as "a whitened sepulcher"—good-looking on the outside, but rotten on the inside.

Like an ear of corn, I had the sensation of layer after layer being stripped away faster than my body, or even my imagination, could restore the damage and regenerate.

It seemed that being a patient was bad for my morale and my physical well-being. I began to understand what Dr. Mosser meant during our earlier conversations, when he asked me about including my family for emotional support during the treatment process. "This treatment is a different level of things," he cautioned.

During the three years, hospitalization was considered again, but during the previous hospitalization, I was bored and behaved like a child. For example, at lunchtime, when peas were served, I would put a green pea in a spoon and use the spoon like a slingshot to shoot at targets on the wall.

Yet through three years of illness, I identified a set of eclectic rules to help me through situations. Some rules applied to my relationship with doctors—develop a good rapport with your physician; never break an appointment lest the physician think you're not taking treatment seriously; and do not second-guess the physician. Personal rules included—impose self-discipline; do not develop destructive behaviors like skipping meals or sleep; learn to be tough minded; challenge yourself; and help others.

For me, teaching was my best therapy and was the most constructive outlet for getting the creative juices to flow, to develop new interests, and to concentrate on tasks outside of self—like writing, sketching, photography, attending dramatic and musical events, and modeling.

For several months, for example, I was the prima modela who sat for the sculpting of three bronze heads by Minnesota sculptor, Alonzo Hauser. One head is now at the Walker Art Center in Minneapolis, and the collection is housed at Macalester College in St Paul, Minnesota. Under Hauser's tutelage, I learned to see things anew and to create art in three rather than two dimensions. Often when occupied creatively, I forgot about myself and I transcended physical problems. Artistic endeavors were akin to ascending to the top of the water tower and feeling the wind blow new ideas.

The radiation therapy for Hodgkin's Disease from 1958 to 1961 spanned my maturing years, from age twenty-three to twenty-six. During that period, each successive radiation set was of shorter duration. Each year after 1961 I underwent a thorough evaluation of the status of my Hodgkin's Disease. After about a decade of followup, Dr. Mosser concluded that, although the disease had been arrested, it was not cured. In the dawn of radiation treatment of Hodgkin's disease, I was placed in the third classification of treatment results, that is, alive ten to twenty years after initial diagnosis.

Chapter Three:

Early Physicians

First Resident, Dr. Lundeen (1958)

I sought new friendships, but for five years, I lived my life alone. I had rebuffed my family, so it was unavailable to me. My colleagues were occupied with their careers, the sorority sisters constituted a clique who did not welcome newcomers, and the other patients were dissimilar to me in age and education. But, a hospital coffee shop, situated midway between the hospital and the sorority house, provided an outlet to meet new people. I decided that after my early morning radiation treatments, I would stop for a cup of coffee and a bagel to meet the attractive residents, who seemed engaged in interesting conversations until I walked through the revolving door of the coffee shop. Then the room became silent. I believe that the residents were talking about me. The next day, I asked Dr. Mosser about the talk in the coffee shop, and not at all surprised, he replied, "To the immature, you are an anathema. Some 'docs' think you're a tragic beauty soon to die. It's simply hospital gossip." I sat alone for several more weeks, but one day, Dr. Bruce Lundeen, the resident for my case, joined my table, ordered coffee and a roll, and began to converse. His presence at my table encouraged other residents and doctors to join me on future days. The gossip about me subsided and my condition was perceived as less threatening each day. They were aware that they also could be stricken with Hodgkin's Disease.

It is true that I met interesting residents at the coffee shop, but a cup of coffee each morning was an insufficient stimulus to occupy my day in my battle of illness. The hospital was on a university campus and adjacent to it was the psychology building where I poked my head into a classroom one day and wondered if I should enroll in courses. When I consulted Dr. Mosser, he suggested that I wait for the new quarter until I felt physically stronger and could work toward a degree. I conceded, but each day, when I returned to the sorority house, I passed the magnificent Gothic building on the corner that housed the English Department.

One day in 1961, I walked into the building to investigate the courses, but this time, without discussing options with Dr. Mosser, I sat in on a class, disregarding registration, reasoning that an additional student would make little difference. Distinguished poets like Allen Tate, Robert Penn Warren, Robert Frost, and others of their ilk taught the summer sessions at the University of Minnesota. I audited Allen Tate's poetry class, wearing a black, summer-weight jacket with a hood to cover my collection of scars and marks. Professor Tate, always nattily dressed, routinely entered class drinking a carton of chocolate milk and wearing a light blue and white seersucker, pin striped summer suit with a blue shirt. When he finished the milk, he set his carton on the desk and began to instruct formally or informally about his favorite poets—Ezra Pound, T. S. Eliot, Robert Frost, Marianne Moore, Edna St. Vincent Millay, Emily Dickinson, and other renowned American poets. Although I was not enrolled, I wanted Professor Tate to criticize an essay assignment he required of the other students attending his class. When leaving class the day the assignment was due, I dropped my essay in his out-basket like the other students.

The next day, after he finished his chocolate milk, Professor Tate called my name and asked me to stand. I was convinced of a reprimand, or at the very least to be asked to leave class. Instead, Professor Tate smiled and delivered a flattering appraisal of my essay on *The Painted Head.*[2] He asked me to read the essay aloud in class. Since I was without a voice and could not read aloud, I asked his indulgence. He read it in his wonderful Southern accent. The other students now wanted to meet and talk with me. I was the new kid on the block unfamiliar to them before, but now I had something to offer.

I registered for English classes at the University of Minnesota and began my master's degree, which I completed in the next two years. I was eager to use the prime years of my life productively although illness was taking its toll. As I told Dr. Mosser, "I can wear my scars publicly if I am productive." He agreed, helped me with my enrollment, and arranged for the cancellation of all my school fees.

Dr. Mosser not only helped me academically, but he

---

[2] The Painted Head is a poem by John Crowe Ransom about a metaphoric head that fell on the floor and cracked.

also offered advice socially. He was the person who suggested that I accept social invitations. One such invitation was to go sailing on Lake Minnetonka with Dr. Lundeen. When Dr. Lundeen phoned to invite me to go sailing the following Sunday, I knew I would accept. I was ready to crew, which I had not done for several years. I bought a new purple angora bathing suit to lessen the contrast with my scarred body, and wore my usual man's white shirt with a pair of white slacks, a sailor hat, and my old white sneakers. I offered to pack a picnic basket for four people because Dr. Lundeen invited another doctor and his wife to join us. In his blue Corvette convertible, Bruce Lundeen drove Dr. and Mrs. Warner and me to Lake Minnetonka, one of Minnesota's larger and more beautiful lakes. For the first time in months, I remembered what feeling normal was like. I was not well, but I realized that I was getting healthier. We docked the boat on the wharf, rigged it, and sailed gloriously until lunchtime and moored at a restaurant on the lakeshore to buy beverages for lunch. The lakeside restaurant was filled by the usual large Sunday gathering of yachtsmen. Just when we planned to dock the boat by the restaurant, a gust of wind blew strongly, causing the mainsail to come about and dramatically knock the skipper into the water in front of everyone. A good sailor, Dr. Lundeen was rather embarrassed and was displeased with the way we crewed. The people from the restaurant laughed uproariously and applauded, but some helped Bruce climb out of the water and turn the boat topside. They too were surprised by the mishap. It wasn't funny, but it was the first time I laughed in a long while!

Dr. Lundeen surprised me with an invitation to go

sailing again the next Sunday. He cared about me as a patient and was becoming a steady friend in my life on Sunday afternoons. After years of solitary Sundays, sailing and meeting new people filled the summer months with release and pleasure. He became interested in me romantically and considered Hodgkin's Disease an irrelevant disease. I was nearing the five-year survival mark on the bell curve.

To my surprise, my oldest sister, Linda, invited Dr. Lundeen to visit at her lake house in northern Minnesota and found him to be an impressive gentleman. An only son of a Virginian mother, his demeanor and mannerisms were Southern. Dr. Mosser, Dr. Lundeen's other social promoter, gave some interesting advice, "You know," he said, "There are worse things that can happen in marriage besides death."

Prior to dating Dr. Lundeen, my social life had been stunted by illness. At age twenty-five, I still felt too immature to make a significant decision about marriage. My friends were being married, which was motivating, but I remained indecisive.

Physicians' Open House

Dr. Lundeen and I were invited to an open house hosted by two doctors. The hosts held the party in their basement. Ironically, I eventually married one of the hosts. As I stood at the top of the stairs and looked down, I could see one of the party's hosts, a doctor I had been observing at the hospital coffee shop for several months. He wore a mustard-colored shirt, which his large, black olive eyes accented and evoked an ancient motif that captured my imagination. I looked forward to meeting this tall, thin, dark man who resembled my grandfather. At the coffee shop, I would stop and pet Bruno, his dog.

"It is nice to meet you finally," he said at the party. "You are very welcome, and we wish you well." It was a great opening for what I anticipated was going to be a boring party.

Being in the hospital environment permitted me to meet the kind of men I wanted to know. I made a decision to date physicians only. I began to reflect on dating seriously. I considered the pros and cost of marriage.

Chapter Four:

The Family

The Family Excludes Itself from My Recovery

Neither my parents nor my siblings were engaged in my recovery. I can't remember informing them about my illness. I believe I actually excluded them. With the exception of my youngest sister, no one in my family visited me during the first treatment period. Maybe it was my mother's stoic attitude toward illness that caused our lack of communication or the embarrassment I caused her by being ill. My father respected and was proud of me until I became ill, and then all attention ceased and like Mother, he remained aloof. I actually expected an occasional visit from them, and I was surprised and hurt when my parents did not inquire about my health. My family's absence might have been the result of my independence. I abided by the family mantra—"Do not complain; nobody is listening."

It is true that my three older siblings were pursuing careers and at the same time, two were mothers of young children. I did regret, however, the absence of a short visit or a phone call. My doctors often asked about my family, but I had no answers. Embarrassed about their behavior, I often lied about their whereabouts. Out of habit, I became a secretive and private person who learned to explain little. Nonetheless, I needed and wanted my family's emotional and moral support, even if I did not know how to obtain it. Their absence made me feel abandoned and forlorn. In a real and an existential sense, I created a life to live alone.

Only once during these four years did a family member, my youngest sister, visit me. One afternoon, after I had slept for three days without awakening, my little sister made a surprise visit. She was unfamiliar about how to enter the sorority house for the first visit. She didn't know that guests entered through the main door, accessible by contacting the housemother, who owned the only master key. The housemother had Wednesdays off, which was the day Karen visited. Karen was a resourceful person, but was unable to contact the housemother, so she scaled the three story, red brick wall by climbing from one patio-like porch to the next. She awakened me by scratching on the third floor screen window of my bedroom. Non-sorority sisters had to live on the top floor. When Karen awakened me, I was happy to realize I maintained my sense of humor and teased her, "I, Rapunzel, cannot let down my hair because I have none." Karen crawled in the window and we sat on the sunny patio and chatted. I was delighted to see her and happy to know that we were able to laugh about my appearance. My loss of hair and purple neck made me look like a skinned turkey, but my sister had fortuitously purchased a plaid sports cap for me. She also brought a copy of a prayer entitled "A Hodgkin's Patient," which she said Mother preserved in her prayer book and recited daily.

The Family Crosses the Ocean from
Vienna to Montana

At age eight, when I first visited Helena, where Mother was born, I wondered what compelled her parents to journey from Vienna, Austria over the Atlantic Ocean and travel half-way across the United States to Montana in the 1880s. It is true that silver mining lured the fictional Dan Cody of *The Great Gatsby* fame, as well as many immigrants westward to Montana, but my grandfather did not work in the silver mines; did not work at the large off-sale liquor store he owned; and did not work anywhere else, for that matter.

In my few conversations about grandfather's childhood, he did not respond to my inquiries about his origins, but pulled my braids and smiled when I introduced the subject of his background. I had no facts and could not derive answers from what little my grandfather, my mother, aunts, and uncles revealed about their travels to America or their early years in the United States. The silence about the family's landing in the United States and the vagaries about the family's early life in Montana remained a secret.

I visited Helena several times and plagued grandfather to open grandmother's two large storage trunks on the third floor of the Helena home. I thought the trunks might hold some valuable secrets. When we opened the trunks, I found only old photos, antique watches, and music records that were perforated around the edges. When we played the records on the old wind-up phonograph, they were reminiscent of the music from The Third Man. Sadly, when grandfather and I touched the rolls and rolls of beautiful, old Viennese lace, the remnants decomposed. The trunks revealed no answers to my questions about the Screnar heritage. I continued to search for grandfather's Jewish origins. When we closed the trunks, I felt as if we ended the story of the grandmother I never met.

At two different times in my adult life, I visited Vienna to search for available records about the Screnar heritage. The name had been anglicized, so it was difficult to trace. After serious investigations, I was unable to discover the original spelling, and the searches proved fruitless. Despite the fact that we were raised Christian, with little reason I was convinced of grandfather's Jewish heritage. It was then that I decided to study Judaism and convert to the religion in order to carry on what I deduced was my family heritage. Since I decided my heritage was Jewish, I undertook Jewish studies, converted to Judaism in my early twenties, eventually married a Jewish man, and lived a Jewish life.

After the death of grandmother, grandfather paid little attention to his family and gave no advice to my mother or her siblings. Mother told me that her father confessed that since he was no longer a husband, he no longer felt like a father. It was one of the few revelations Mother made about her family.

Tall, thin, and an extremely handsome older man, my grandfather was a well-groomed gentleman in the European style. He usually wore beige corduroy trousers, white French cuffed shirts, and tweed jackets with suede patches on the elbows. I often observed him reading German newspapers. My oldest sister insisted that grandfather spoke German only. I was equally persuaded that he spoke to me in English. Otherwise, how did we communicate?

Grandfather had thick steel gray hair that turned silver as he aged, which matched his steel blue eyes. He was a quiet man of few words whom I loved to visit and with whom I held a strong inexplicable emotional and physical affinity. Throughout my life, I was in perpetual search of my grandfather's alter ego. My psychiatrist informed me that grandchildren do not have an Oedipal complex with a grandparent, but I was convinced he was wrong because I had something akin to it.

Mother was a stoic person and a classic beauty whose appearance resembled her father. She had thick, silver hair and steel blue eyes, accented by high cheekbones. I was unable to discover the roots of her stoic behavior, but attributed its origin to grandmother's premature death when Mother was a youngster. The resulting grief seemed never to dissipate. Mother's behavior also was formed by a harsh past about which she rarely spoke and never complained. She was the daughter of a widowed immigrant father and a mother who died at a young age. Named Maryanne, Mother was the first-born and became the surrogate parent of two brothers, John and Joseph, and two sisters, Anne and Frances. Her oldest brother became a businessman and her youngest brother was a professional baseball player. Mother became a volunteer teacher, Anne a state senator, and Frances declared no profession. Her siblings pursued different professions, and all developed successful careers. As immigrants, the family was rejected by the society in which they lived, but they overcame the rejection, worked their way through school, and found niches in society for themselves, even as misfits. They were physically attractive young adults of character and strength.

Screnar-Kirchner Lineage

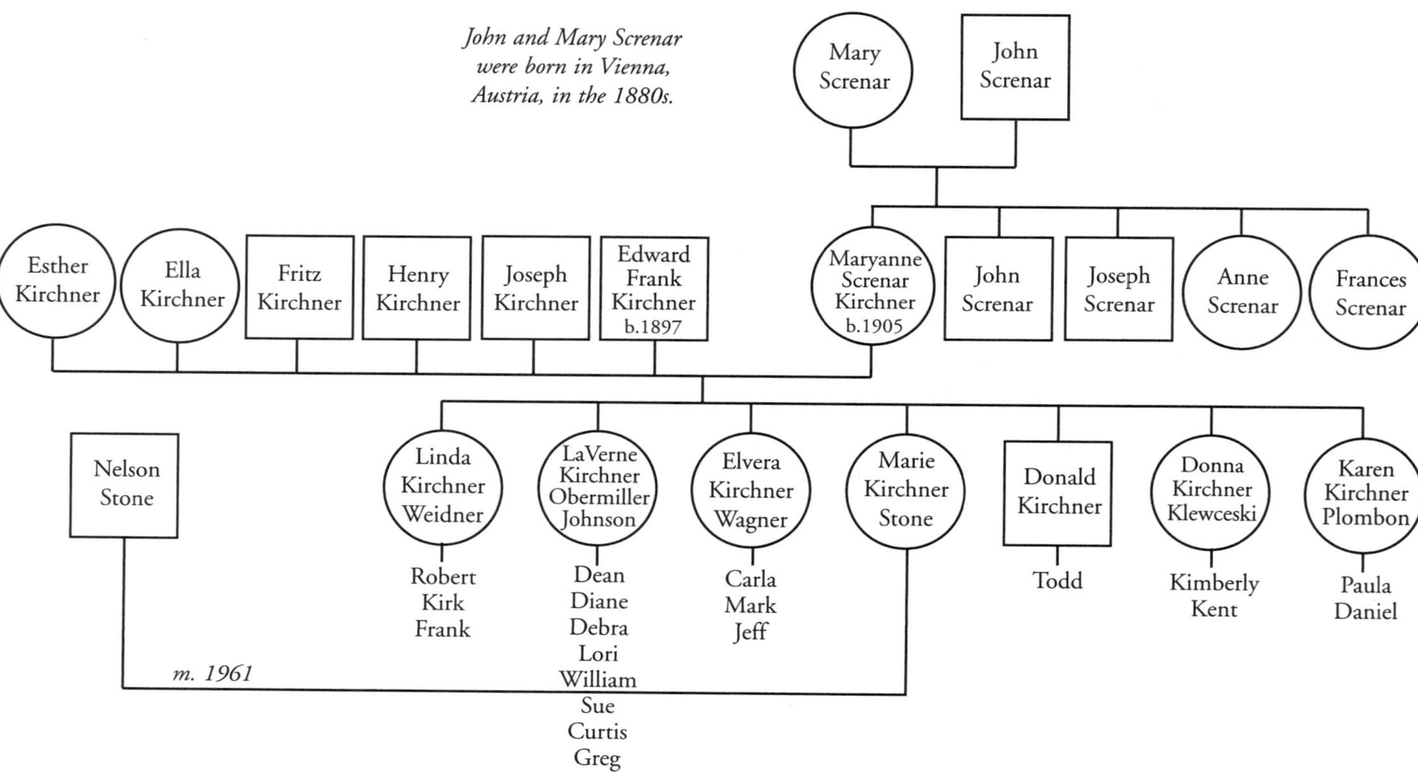

Mother was a strong person who established the emotional tone in both her father's and her new husband's homes. Her behavior was erratic and no one could guess what the tone might be. She might be mouse quiet one minute, whistle a merry tune the next, and then shout angrily. Our father followed her lead, as he was wont to do in most things.

Mother rejected illness, perhaps because of the illness her mother suffered, which the doctor labeled cancer. Mother objected to any child in the family becoming sick, and when someone did, she inadvertently instilled guilt as if somehow the person was to blame. Mother also rejected us when we had physical accidents, which caused us to camouflage our injuries.

When I finally told Mother I had Hodgkin's Disease and that I planned to deal with it through help from my physician, she stoically accepted the diagnosis and readily agreed to be excluded. I didn't tell her that Dr. Mosser insisted that she and Dad see him. Although Mother exempted herself from the problems incumbent with my having Hodgkin's Disease, I felt that she cared deeply about me, but was unable to express her emotions when it involved illness. My illness caused Mother to be not only stoically silent, but also coolly detached, frustrated, and angered. She played the Pontius Pilate role and washed her hands of the whole matter.

The ultimate result of Mother's stoicism was devastating and manifested itself in the lack of display of physical or emotional affection. She was not demonstrative and did not touch, embrace, or kiss me once in my lifetime. I adored and emulated her and considered myself made in her image and likeness—that is, I mirrored her appearance and copied her style—her propriety, dignity, grace, and her character.

She and I differed emotionally—I was passionate and effusive, the reverse side of her stoicism. The only time she revealed her capacity to express emotional feelings was when she and Dad sat on the sofa evenings after dinner in an amorous fondling. She also expressed sexual passion. For example, one night, a moaning sound emanated from her bedroom. Alarmed, I jumped out of bed and hurried downstairs to see what was wrong. Nothing, however, was wrong. Her moaning was the sound of lovemaking pleasure. I tiptoed back upstairs with increased resolve to make Mother hold me in her arms one day before she died.

Mother could be fun-loving. For instance, she would decorate the dining room table with yellow napkins, daisies, and yellow paper cups to make a gray day sunny and a little brighter. She would bake a chocolate cake and invite my friends to join in a party on Sunday afternoons. Mother used other devices like having us dress in costumes some evenings to perform a play. Other nights, she would push aside the dining room table and teach us how to dance waltzes, the foxtrot, or the jitterbug. Her passions were hidden unless she was upset, when she readily revealed her frustration and anger. For example, after my sister and I washed dishes, Mother would inspect each newly wiped glass in the cupboard by holding the glass to the light at the rim and the base to check if it showed water spots. If so, we had to re-wash the glasses again and again until she was satisfied.

I think it was the influence of Montana that made Mother an environmentalist of sorts. We children had to turn off the lights when a room was empty, regulate the water from the faucet when we were brushing our teeth, and control the heat to below normal temperature. She had other rules to save the environment. For instance, during World War II, Mother and the family hiked to the fields to fill gunny sacks of milk weed pods so the government could manufacture parachutes for the air force.

Noted for managing an orderly and spotless home, every drawer from the kitchen to the bedrooms was organized, and all articles were logically placed for ease of locating them efficiently. Our clothing reflected the cleanliness of the house; we were always attired neatly. Mother forbade our leaving the house with wrinkled jeans or messy hair. A hard working person, Mother was resourceful and frugal.

When she volunteered as a teacher at a nearby elementary school, she often invited the poor children from the school to our home for lunch. If she invited too many students and lunch was scarce on that day, Mother had a good trick. She invented the story that her own children were spoiled and refused to eat the good food she was serving because they were fussy eaters. Mother winked at us with delight in telling the fib to the students. In reality, we were famished for lunch, as well as for the affection she so lavishly bestowed upon her students. These were Mother's favorite days, but we disliked it when our cheese sandwiches and soup were devoured by others.

Father was a completely different kind of person from Mother. Mother's stoicism contrasted Father's casual approach to life. A fun-loving and handsome man, Dad exuded success and confidence, smiling at everyone easily. He possessed color crayon blue eyes that twinkled readily when he laughed, which he did often. He was appreciative of the good relationships he had with his siblings and his many friends and acquaintances.

Parents Marry and Move from Montana to Minnesota

At age twenty-five, when he moved to Montana from Minnesota, Dad courted several ladies in addition to Mother. One woman audaciously followed him from Helena to St. Cloud, causing a great rift in our house with unending verbal repercussions. She had been Mother's best girlfriend in Helena, and Father clandestinely promised to marry each of them. I understood Mother's wrath about her husband and her friend.

At home, Father possessed autocratic tendencies, and his directives underscored Mother's stern supervision. Jointly, their discipline, order, and the consequences for misbehavior superceded their love and affection. For example, dinner was a ritual, which Father wanted served promptly at six o'clock each evening in the dining room. It made no difference if someone waited all week for a boy to phone to ask for a long awaited date. The telephone was off limits at dinner hour. Additionally, each person was assigned to select and discuss a topic of interest for one night a week, Monday through Friday evenings. The topics varied from current events to school issues, but frequently, other concerns replaced these discussions.

Dad usually spoke politely, but at times he reverted to sarcastic remarks, which he said with a smirk on his face. For instance, if he thought a dress more appropriate for an occasion when I was wearing jeans, he would say with sarcasm, "Poor, unattractive Maria. She has only boy's clothing to wear." To my oldest sister, his sarcasm often focused on her career about which he would snidely remark, "A nursing career isn't good enough for Linda. She insists on working for a salary." He displayed the most sarcasm to Donna for what he called, "Not living up to Maria's standards." In fact, she surpassed them, but he was adroit at pointing his blunt remarks for effect, and we dared not respond.

The Great Depression forced Father to change from one occupation to another. Formally uneducated, he was an intellectually capable man with skilled hands. Before he left for Montana to work in the silver mines, he had begun a start-up construction company in Minnesota, which developed into a large housing development. He had been a successful entrepreneur with his brothers and wanted to repeat this success when he returned from Montana. Mother, however, wanted financial security and encouraged him to become employed by a company that provided it. Father accepted her advice and took a position with the Great Northern Railroad, about which he often complained bitterly. Some days he would arrive home from work with a newspaper article excerpted from *The New York Times*, dealing with the construction of public works during the Great Depression. He insisted on our listening throughout dinner to his tirade, "This is what I should be doing. I could build these government projects as well as anyone and make more money at one job than I earn all year." A week or so later, a different newspaper article would provoke him to reiterate the same harangue about managing road or bridge construction. It was his frustration over the growing success of the housing industry that occurred in the aftermath of World War II that caused him to slam his fist on the table and announce that he refused to waste his life at his present job. His verbal effusion often overrode the topics we had been assigned to discuss at the dinner table. Interestingly, he never raised his voice at Mother or held her accountable for his problems. With her, he was always a polite gentleman.

Mother met Father, Edward Frank Kirchner, in Helena, Montana, but he was born in 1897 in Richmond, a small town in Minnesota. He departed to work in the silver mines of Montana for a season at age twenty-five. He was eight years Mother's senior. Soon after he met Mother, he courted and married her. Following their wedding, Father and his new wife moved to St. Cloud, Minnesota, a small city one hour north of Minneapolis. St. Cloud was a tidy middle class city with a population of 50,000 people, mostly of German descent. Because it was built on the banks of the Mississippi River, St. Cloud became a major transportation hub, transporting grain, wood, and other raw materials. Farming in the outlying areas encouraged the flour milling industry and forestry promoted the paper mill industry. Granite deposits resulted in the development of the granite crusher industry, another major occupation and source of wealth for the city. The city grew in prosperity and population.

Education was a mainstay in this central Minnesota town because of the presence of a Benedictine monastery. By the turn of the century, two Benedictine single sex universities had been built in the outlying area of the city, and at the end of World War II, the state college, now university, and two major high schools had been constructed in the heart of the city. As the decades passed, the city expanded southward along the banks of the Mississippi

River to become like a suburb of Minneapolis. The St. Cloud citizens objected vehemently because they wanted to maintain the quality of the smaller city.

Mother appreciated living in a city this size, although she was isolated from her family in Montana. The city was neat, prosperous, and beautiful. The shifting job market during the Great Depression caused the citizens' socio-economic statuses to be in flux. We were middle class, and luxuries were not part of our repertoire. I had to finance my own college tuition, earn spending money, buy my own clothing, and pay for all necessities except food and shelter. At times, we ate what Mother called "healthy meals," consisting solely of vegetables from the garden because they were nutritious and economical. Dessert was a rarity unless Mother baked. Drinking soda was unheard of except for Dad's occasional purchase of a six-pack of Ginger Ale.

The Kirchner Family Experiences Serious Illnesses

During the Depression, in addition to his main job, Dad held two other positions, city assessor and bowling alley manager. Like his brothers, our father also was an effective business entrepreneur. Together, they developed a pharmacy, a bowling alley, a funeral home, a restaurant and cocktail bar, and a housing development. These four brothers and their two sisters cooperated with each other and formed a tightly knit corps that enabled them to manage their successful business ventures. Father's family also knew how to enjoy life and each other. They spent happy days together as outdoorsmen, fishing for walleyes and bass in one of Minnesota's ten thousand lakes, and hunting pheasants in the fields with their prize dog, Curly.

Socially conscious, they applied their building craft and talent by joining with other community members to construct housing for poor families.

Health was one gift denied the Kirchner family. Typical for this era, three brothers died before the age of sixty from different kinds of cancer, as did their youngest sister, Esther. The most dapper son, Henry, committed suicide, reminiscent of Edwin Arlington Robinson's poem, "Richard Corey":

> *He was a gentleman from sole to crown . . .*
> *And he was always quietly arrayed.*
> *And admirably schooled in every grace . . .*
> *To make us wish that we were in his place. . . .*
> *And Richard Cory, one calm summer night,*
> *Went home and put a bullet through his head.*

Like so many other events of significance in our family, we did not discuss Uncle Henry's suicide or any illnesses. We cared for our health and did not smoke or drink. Except for suicide, most health problems in the Kirchner family were hereditary. In each of my father's siblings' families, including ours, at least one and sometimes more than one young adult, between ages twenty and forty, died or was taken ill with heart disease or different cancers—leukemia, breast cancer, Hodgkin's Disease, cervical cancer, thyroid and ovarian cancers. Two members suffered from polycythemia vera, and two suffered from strokes. Death was familiar to the family.

In 1961, at the end of my first three years of therapy for Hodgkin's Disease, my brother-in-law was in a coma between December and April, caused by a car accident from which he never recovered. His extended hospitaliza-tion caused Mother to postpone a necessary physical check-up. She was not feeling well and had been suffering from serious stomach pains since before Christmas. She had been diagnosed with gastrointestinal problems, which we thought at most was a gall bladder or a thyroid inflam-mation. She wanted to postpone her hospitalization in order to preserve the holidays and create a grand celebra-tion for my late brother-in-law's children. Mother lived with increasing unuttered pain.

Ironically, the family became less attentive to Mother's illness than to the dying brother-in-law's coma. I chal-lenged the idea of placing greater emphasis on death than on life.

For five months, Mother suffered in silence and refused to enter the hospital until there was some closure to my brother-in-law's coma. After his death in April, Mother entered the hospital with a diagnosed cancer. Her body was already jaundiced. It turned a beautiful golden color and her hair formed a silver crown similar to the regal, entombed Greek goddesses, which she was. During this period, when I felt physically capable, I drove to St. Cloud to visit Mother at first in the hospital and then at home. My older sisters and I helped to care for Mother in the hospital. We oiled her lips and inserted drops of water into her mouth as if she were a bird. We obtained a mobile mattress and tried to provide a supportive emotional struc-ture for her.

After a two-month hospital stay, the doctor told us Mother was dying. She decided to die at home, where my younger siblings took charge, giving her intravenous feed-ings, watering her lips, and caring for as many physical and emotional needs and desires as possible. The older siblings had to tend to their families and their jobs, and I had to return to Minneapolis for more treatments. When Mother came home from the hospital, her most prized friend became Chipper, my little Mexican Chihuahua, whom she surprisingly allowed to roam and romp on her bed. She hugged, petted, and kissed Chipper, and we decided the affection bestowed upon our little dog was a substitute for her expression of feelings toward us. Mother wanted to die and died peacefully at age fifty-seven in July 1961. In our lifetimes, she displayed no emotion or affection for us. Our deep love of her could not triumph over her stoicism.

Mother's Death and Funeral

On her deathbed, I realized even more than I did in life that Mother often and easily broke my heart. Her loneliness and sadness were mine. She lived estranged from her siblings in Montana, who exchanged no more than five visits in thirty years.

Her father never visited, although Mother attended his funeral in Montana. Hers was a sad and unfulfilled life in which she worked selflessly to make a rewarding life for all of us.

I insisted on telephoning her siblings in Montana about her death. Her siblings angered me because of their infrequent visits. Why visit after Mother died? I thought it important to replace the euphemism "She passed away," with brutal frankness, "At two o'clock today, Mother died." Standing in the kitchen hall and telephoning the relatives, I requested her sisters respond actively as they should have when Mother was living. My anger at Mother's relatives, who had visited infrequently when she was alive and attended the funeral, did not subside. After the burial, when they were conversing in the living room, my sister and I, to avoid their presence, went to the kitchen and began washing the stacks and stacks of dirty plates and cups left from the reception after the wake. I was seething and mumbling under my breath when my sister turned to me to explain that I should forget about the insult. I turned and in response, hit my sister across the face with the wet dishcloth, making a huge red mark on her cheek. I deeply regretted such a preposterous gesture. My sister cried and asked if I was trying to make her look like me with a red radiation mark. Then I began to cry, but Mother wasn't present to solve the problem. We walked outside so we could not be heard, and together we cried and cried in the backyard. My sister understood my anger and forgave me.

The visitors from Montana went home after a day, and I never communicated with them again.

On a June afternoon, four years later in 1965, my father, at age sixty-eight, died in bed and was discovered by my niece, who lived close by and often checked on him as he was aging and living alone.

Family in Transition

In our immediate family, the younger and the older siblings did not really know each other well because the seven siblings never lived in one house together. Our ages spanned twenty years. I was the middle sibling dividing the two families—Linda, LaVerne, and Elvera were the older siblings. The twins (Donna and Don), Karen, and I made up the younger group. The older siblings and I were each born three years apart; the twins were five years younger than me; and my baby sister was four years younger than them. Our two-story house was too small, but sufficient room was created when the three older siblings departed for their life's careers when the three younger siblings were growing up. The first floor of the house was made up of a sizeable dining room, a large living room, and a comfortable sized master bedroom for my parents.

We children slept on the second floor where there were three small bedrooms and a hall with a large magnificent pipe organ that dominated the entire space of one wall. The genesis of the organ remained unknown except it was considered a family heirloom and important to Mother, who maintained it in mint condition. All members of the family were interested in music, but they manifested it diversely. My parents sang German songs a cappella, and all siblings sang in the school choir. Everyone in the family played piano and a wind or brass instrument. When I was taking piano and wanted to change to trumpet, I had to wait. Mother's theory was, "You don't have to start again, but you can't quit in the middle." A half-year had to transpire before I could begin trumpet.

I often played in the toy room on the second floor, which my father built under the eaves of the south side of the house. It was a manicured place where Mother organized the toys alphabetically, and we removed and replaced them alphabetically.

During the first five years of my life, I often played alone for hours with my shabby gold and brown teddy bear. I was a tomboy who found pleasure in bears rather than dolls.

In the winter, I went ice-skating, sledding, and tried skiing. In the spring, I played marbles, touch football, tennis, and baseball with the neighborhood boys. Each spring, when the snow thawed, it filled our large garden with water, and my brother and I would rig Dad's cement box, a container for holding quantities of cement mix for construction, as a raft and sailed across the garden. If either of the participants moved too spasmodically, we'd capsize. It was usually I who fell in. One afternoon, I intentionally threw my brother into the cold water to soak him as I had been soaked. After that episode, we were forbidden to play Huckleberry Finn, which is what we called the garden game.

In the hot summer months, I went for a swim in the quarry where I dived from the tall, steep straight cliffs suspended ten to twenty-five feet above the water level. The quarries were deep spring-fed holes filled with one hundred or more feet of clear blue water, resulting from the removal of granite. I could recite "Kubla Khan" as I dived into the water from the highest cliff and watched my shadow descend and be devoured by the water. My goal was to capture the gold bottle caps that remained visible as I threw them into the water in advance of my dive. The bottle caps could be seen until they were about fifteen feet deep, where everything below the water turned totally black and nothing could be seen. It was as Ralph Ellison wrote in *Invisible Man*, "The blackness of black." At times, out of breath because I remained deep under water for too long, I became frightened and surfaced as rapidly upward as I could in search of the sunlight, which converted the black water to blue. St. Cloud was the granite capital of the world, so there were a number of quarries where one could swim. One time, when I frightened myself totally and thought that I would not have enough air to ascend to the surface, I promised myself it was my finale and I would dive no more. I resorted to diving from ten-foot diving boards in the city pool when money permitted.

To replace high diving that summer, I began a new project—collecting bugs from the shores of the Mississippi River. Some I kept alive in a series of jelly jars, which I identified, and others I preserved in formaldehyde. Mother disliked the presence of bugs, dead or alive, in her pristine house, so I exchanged the entire collection of some thirty thoughtfully collected specimens with a boy from school, who in turn taught me how to water ski on the Mississippi River.

My three older siblings referred to me as the spoiled kid because I had been the baby of the family for five years, but the name accrued no special favors. In fact, no one in our house could be called spoiled because discipline and character-building superceded pleasure and affection. Whether we were age ten or twenty, Mother held the same expectations for all.

The birth of twins transformed the reference to me as spoiled. I had difficulty analyzing the reason my parents decided to have three more children after me. Perhaps they were concerned about carrying on our heritage with so many other Kirchner relatives dead prematurely. Maybe it was because they liked children and wanted a large family. Or, it could be as simple as liking sex and neglecting birth control. I can remember the shock when late one June afternoon, Mother walked into the house carrying twins in her arms. The boy, Don, was wrapped in a blue blanket and the girl, Donna, in a pink blanket. I am sure my older siblings were aware, but I missed Mother's pregnancy entirely. She was naturally thin and didn't show her pregnancy even when carrying twins. My oldest sister's pregnancies were similar in that she also remained slim. Mother dealt with pregnancy privately in the same manner she did illness. New babies were neither a problem nor a joy. There were no hugs and kisses, no showing off the babies, no cooing and fawning. My first conscious memory of the twins was a photograph of Donna holding a pink angel food cake and Don a blue frosted devil's food cake.

The younger set of children became its own self-reliant unit. I taught them to play tennis, volleyball, and other outdoor sports with the kids in the neighborhood. Our older siblings spoke about the fun they had with our parents—dancing, bowling, picnicking, going out for family dinners, driving to my uncle's lake house for family reunions, helping to build a cottage on an island for my father's nephew, or traveling on the Great Northern Railway to Helena, Montana. The younger siblings replicated few of these activities because my parents weren't as involved with the younger set, which was too young to attend concerts or the movies, go hiking or bowling, or indulge in the activities the older siblings enjoyed.

I spent time searching for new adventures. Since my younger siblings were too young, I was secretive about my risky ventures, which didn't involve my younger siblings. In winters, I hooked on to the bumpers of city buses to skid on the icy roadways and arrive at the business section of the city without paying a bus fare. Infatuated with heights, on a dare from a gang of boys, I balanced on the foot-wide handrail of a walking bridge suspended one hundred feet over a highway and walked across the bridge, where falling meant certain death. I wanted the excitement and had little money to pay for safe activities like snow skiing or high diving at the city pool. Free danger became my teenage pastime.

When I was unoccupied in the mornings, Mother assigned work projects, which took away my play time. I had to help Mother in the garden—plant and cultivate potatoes, pick and snap green beans, shell peas, and husk corn so she could preserve these garden vegetables for her "healthy dinners." My experience at home gardening helped me to secure employment at a truck farm three miles from my home. I walked this distance four mornings a week. At the truck farm, I bunched vegetables—green onions, carrots, scallions—or boxed strawberries and seasonal fruits. The old men at the truck farm taught me how to swear in what was referred to as "truck driver's language," which I delighted in using in front of my polite friends.

We seven children constituted two different kinds of families. My younger siblings participated in different activities and parented themselves.

Upon my high school graduation, my older sisters began to make their career decisions. Linda planned to become a nurse in the Navy. I can recall the excitement when the family gathered to sew nametags in the necks of her blouses and on the waistbands of her skirts. I was proud of her. But, alas, she changed her mind. One day, she arrived home from an interview to say that she was going to accept a job as a secretary at an industrial plant that manufactured war materials. Linda, the oldest sibling, was to be the first to attend college, and would set an example for the rest of us. I did however understand her reasons for wanting to earn money, which is always a compelling force in a poor family.

Linda's job decision did result in other long-term positive outcomes. At the company, she met a young, attractive, and capable man who had just returned from the Navy. After a short courtship, she married him and helped to finance his college. I questioned the reasons for financing his college career and not her own, because Linda was brilliant academically. As his wife, she evolved into an astute top-notch business woman, and together, she and her husband built a successful financial empire comprised of several retail stores, an apartment development, a bank, storage units, and the construction of large housing projects in Northern Minnesota, in Canada, and in the Dominican Republic. Linda and her husband, Robert Weidner, also raised three outstanding sons, R.C., Kirk, and Frank, who are now college graduates and businessmen of consequence. Linda continues to regret not having a college degree, but she still manages a business at age seventy-five. Linda has suffered from polycythemia vera for seven years, but it does not curtail her activities or life style.

Illness and death were central to our family's existence, and they taught me about the devastation on the living. The needs of the healthy, it seemed, were subsumed by the needs of the sick. LaVerne, my second oldest sister, married in lieu of attending college. Two major tragedies altered her young life, putting college out of the question. LaVerne's first husband suffered from an automobile accident, which put him in a coma until he died after a six-month hospitalization. His situation made me seriously reflect on the feasibility of mercy killing, fully recognizing its legal ramifications. Sitting in her husband's room on nights when I drove from Minneapolis, I would wait for the "special nurse" on duty to leave for her coffee break, when I considered removing my brother-in-law's suction tube. I could not muster the courage, but I did ask myself, "What is the purpose of living a comatose life when death is imminent?"

After several years passed, LaVerne met and married a man who bore a great resemblance to her first husband. Our family was excited to see our sister ensconced in a good relationship again. When she married, she had three of her own children, four of her husband's offspring, and an eighth child they bore together. She developed the eight children into a remarkable, cohesive strong family unit. All attended college—two in healthcare majors and the others in engineering, computers, and design majors. LaVerne demanded that her siblings treat all of her children equally. In fact, we had to give presents to all eight children or none could be given at all. Her second husband built a large, lovely split-level home on the Mississippi River, sodded the acre-large front yard, built a pool, and planted flowers throughout the yard. One spring day, the waves moved forcefully down the Mississippi River, making torpedoes of tree trunks and flooding the bottom floor of the house. The family saw the power of Mother Nature wiping out all in her path. As the water became dangerously high, the Red Cross phoned and insisted the family evacuate.

My three younger siblings and my father were living in our birth house, but they accommodated LaVerne's family, who moved into the house. My sister's husband re-built a more magnificent house than the original, and the family returned to living in harmony for several years. However, tragedy struck again when her second husband was diagnosed with mesothelioma, or asbestos poisoning, which he probably contracted on his prolonged voyages serving in World War II on naval submarines. Her husband suffered agonizing pain. The family learned about the use of alternative medicine—biofeedback, yoga, acupuncture, health food, and other techniques. Holistic and Western medicine did not solve the problem.

Their eight children and my sister mutually agreed to stop all life support systems and let her husband and their father die peacefully. She lost two husbands and her home, yet my sister never complained. LaVerne taught me how to bear hardship.

Elvera, my third sister, who suffered from flu-like symptoms that plagued her early life, grew out of them. She became a florist and especially enjoyed making corsages from day-old flowers and delivering them to the elderly and sick people at hospitals and churches. She made corsages for those who otherwise could not afford to buy flowers. She married an ex-Marine and raised a family of three children—daughter Carla, who became a nurse, and two sons, Mark and Jeff, who graduated with degrees in economics. At her annual check-up at age fifty, the gynecologist diagnosed Elvera with a virulent breast cancer. She went to the hospital for surgery, but after two months, returned home to die with all members of her family present. It was strange, but she craved strawberry floats, which we delivered to her. We learned the value of little simple requests. Elvera was so young, vital, and generous; her death was shockingly unfair.

My two younger sisters, Donna and Karen, my

brother, Don, and I were the first to attend college. The girls went into the healthcare field, and Don pursued news-paper advertising and commercial writing. Don married and fathered a set of twins, who died as infants from heart conditions, and a son, Tim, who also died in infancy. These losses were overwhelming. He became the father of one son, Todd, our only Kirchner namesake, who graduated with a master's degree in business from the University of Minnesota.

Don, at age sixty-two, struggles with polycythemia vera, the same disorder as our older sister, Linda. Polycythemia only rarely afflicts two members of the same family.

Don's twin sister, Donna, while simultaneously working in the healthcare field, became the mother of Kim, a stockbroker, and Kent, a builder. Donna is now divorced from her husband, Frank Klewceski. My youngest sister, Karen, also pursued the healthcare field. A sledding accident in childhood that caused us great concern did not impair her ability to bear children. Our worries and anxieties were in vain. She married Leon Plombon and bore two children; Paula, who became a psychologist, and Daniel, a realtor.

Just as offspring often follow their parents into the same vocation, so too it might be concluded that children who live with family illness often select healthcare as their vocations.

Chapter Five:

Education

Imagination Solves Problems:
Elementary Grades—1940–1945

Early on school mornings, Mother awakened my older sister, Elvera, and me with the greeting, "Wake up, the world's on fire." My sister and I came bounding down the stairs lured by the aroma of Mother's homemade, caramel cinnamon rolls, which she served with succulent orange slices. My eight-year-old sister, who was in the third grade, and I walked to school together each day. I began kindergarten in 1940 at age five. After breakfast, we took turns standing on a kitchen stool so Mother could pleat our thick blonde braids tightly in double pigtails. We usually left home early, skipping happily to school. I goaded my sister to keep my pace whether she felt well or not, and frequently she did not. Mother always warned against running and skipping, but I was a rule breaker.

As soon as the janitor opened the school door, I shot into the classroom so I could study from the geography book that lay open on the round table in the back of the classroom. I was intrigued with the maps and examined them daily, promising myself to visit every country in the world one day. When bored with the regular lessons, I took imaginary journeys to the different lands I discovered on the maps. On weekends, I packed my book bag with travel books checked out from the school library to read at home. One weekend, I read about the Belgian Congo and the next weekend, I read about the Philippine Islands. There was no pattern to my selections except I liked the stories about the ornately dressed colored children— African American, Indians, Asians—and created a photo collection of them and the places they lived. I cut the photos from *National Geographic* and other magazines, which neighbors and friends gave to me or I borrowed from the doctor's office.

In kindergarten, when the first lesson of the day began at nine o'clock, I had to close the geography book and go to my desk. Throughout the elementary grades, by ten o'clock on many mornings, the nurse knocked on the door, interrupting class to signal the teacher to excuse me so I could walk home with my sister, who suffered from stomach pains and headaches, which caused dizziness. I didn't want to miss class, so I rushed Elvera home, six blocks from school or a five-minute round trip for me. I felt sad for my sister, but when we arrived home, I shoved her in the back entrance of our house and slammed the screen door after her. I then rushed back to school to avoid Mother's grimace, which intimated that it was my fault my sister was sick again. When I returned to school, I always felt guilty because I was well and my sister was sick. In later years, I frequently re-experienced this guilt when I became ill myself.

Elementary school was a joy. I especially liked being involved with projects. In the first grade, I remember waving my hand vigorously in class volunteering to read the passage or the story of the day aloud to the other students. Oral readings in class began with fairy tales in the first grade, then advanced to other English narratives, and by third grade, we read Greek myths. When we were reading the Greek myths, I asked the teacher if I could teach the geography of Greece using the atlas from kindergarten. She granted permission, resulting in the third grade teacher's invitation to me to teach part of the third grade class. From 11:30 A.M. to 12:00 P.M. two days a week, the third graders alternated recess and my Greek geography class. This introduction to teaching was the origin of a long and pleasurable career as an educator.

When I was in fourth grade, my health and my sister Elvera's reversed. One late October afternoon, I arrived home early from school with a serious case of the flu. The nurse called to inform my mother that the flu season was causing pupil absences and cautioned bed and liquids. Because I had a 104-degree temperature, my mother put me in her bed and darkened the bedroom so I could sleep. The autumn leaves had just fallen from the trees in both the back and front yards, and the entire family was outside raking and burning leaves. Over the crackling fire, I could hear the loud gleeful voices of my siblings, which made me yearn to join the family in the yard. The high fever caused me to hallucinate and demanded bed rest. As I was resting, class lessons began to merge with the bonfire sounds from outside that evening. We fourth graders had been studying about Thanksgiving pilgrims, who came to my bedroom, where they grew larger than life. The pilgrims were wearing long black dresses and white bonnets and carrying pouches over their shoulders as they marched across Mother's bed. The silhouettes kept chasing me, and I cried out for help. Elvera responded and came into the bedroom from outside. She now treated me irreverently, the same way I had treated her when she became sick in school. She threw Mother's woolen blanket over my head as if to suffocate me, saying spitefully, "Now you know what it feels like to be sick." Finally, the pilgrims stopped their trek westward across my quilt under which I shivered. I had missed my favorite autumn celebration, a bonfire of pungent leaves, which I cherished more than the pumpkins of Halloween or the turkey of Thanksgiving.

After missing several school days, I eagerly returned to classes to learn that the fourth graders were still studying about Thanksgiving. When our fourth grade teacher asked a student to volunteer to draw a Thanksgiving mural on the bulletin board, I gladly offered. Already, I had the images in my mind. I translated the pilgrims from my nightmare into a large Thanksgiving mural, which I drew on brown wrapping paper and tacked to the wall. I developed the habit of interchanging fantasy and reality. When I was sick, the interchange became my escape from reality.

To my great pleasure, the curriculum of the fourth grade focused on geography, and the teacher offered us the opportunity to join a world society, where we sent money to save foreign babies. The world society mailed posters, which featured a picture of a large tree of life with many branches, where photos of children's faces could be pasted. When people donated money to buy a baby, the society in return sent a cameo photo of the baby to the donor. I hung the poster prominently on the wall in my bedroom and joyfully began to collect the money so I could paste ten cameos to fill the blank spaces on the tree. To earn money that year, I began to baby-sit for the neighbors. To save money, I fasted from candy and sweets, a habit I maintain today. I did favors for neighbors to raise nickels and dimes. The number of cameos of babies multiplied on my family tree, but it took me several years to fill all the spaces. I planned to meet the children I "saved" when I eventually traveled to their different countries. Geography, my favorite subject, opened the windows of the world for me.

In the spring of my fifth grade year, illness again struck our household. This time it was my oldest sister, Linda, who at nineteen contracted scarlet fever, resulting in a six-week quarantine for all of the family. Mother insisted that we spend our days around the dining room table learning our school lessons, which Linda was to conduct. The schedule included mathematics from 8:30 to 10:00 in the morning, history and geography were the concentration from 10:30 until noon, and language and reading were the afternoon focus. Everyone had to adjust her classroom materials to make them appropriate for the lesson. Linda was a taskmaster, but it was Mother's rule, "all lessons must be completed whether well or sick," that prevailed. Father's task was to obtain the lessons and materials from school and correct them before their return. With Mother's stoic attitude toward illness, she neither wished not to be involved, nor did she want to be negative about the scarlet fever quarantine, so she sorted the school materials and cleared the working space each morning. She also made a snack for the afternoon break, which one day included pink and white peppermint candy canes. Frustrated, I sucked the candy stick and audaciously made pink polka dots on the quarantine sign attached to the outside front door. Mother was outraged at my behavior, but was reluctant to punish under the circumstances. I envied my sister lounging in her new cranberry chenille robe looking like Jean Harlow, but that was all I envied. It was going to be a long and lingering six-week introduction to spring, and I abhorred it.

At the onset of the quarantine, I begged the school nurse to permit me to live at her house because I had just been selected for the lead role of the sunflower in the spring play, "The Garden Folly." I needed to remain in school for rehearsals, but no matter how important the role was to me, and it was important enough to ask a favor from the nurse, I couldn't break the nurse's will. I did, however, extract her promise that if I returned to school on time for the performance, she would save the part for me. Six weeks later, I surprised the cast and arrived on the stage fully clothed in my costume. The nurse wiggled out of her promise with a new plan when I returned. "We'll pull straws," she said, "and the person who pulls the longer straw, performs." I clenched my eyes and folded my hands, confident I would be chosen because justice was on my side.

Having rehearsed with my sisters' assistance at home, I was a star in "The "Garden Folly," and the cast presented me with one huge sunflower after the performance. Fortunately, after the six-week quarantine, no one else in the family contracted scarlet fever.

Mother sat in the front row, middle section, and applauded politely at the end of each act. After the play, she stood at the end of the hall graciously accepting the compliments about my performance. The other mothers embraced their daughters, but not Mother. Mother let me grapple alone with my conflict about obtaining the part in the play, and she had nothing to say about my performance. But, I know she enjoyed the play.

When I began middle school, I discovered a small library three miles from my home and obtained permission from Mother to walk there after school. In this quaint village library, I discovered the stories of the lives of interesting women. Only after I read a short story by O'Henry, who was writing while in jail, did I realize that real people wrote books. I'm unsure how I thought books were created, but I was surprised to learn this fact so late in life and concluded if real people wrote books, so could I. I decided to write a poem about "a light bulb burning bright, it flickered, and burned out for the night just when it was needed." I submitted the poem to a poetry contest and won a handheld red plastic windmill for first prize. I decided that both the poem and the prize were foolish, and I was embarrassed, so I let the prize sail away with the wind, gave up writing, and returned to reading the biographies about great women like Joan d'Arc, Jane Addams, and Harriett Beecher Stowe.

It was fortuitous, but that spring, the drama coach was casting *Little Women* for the middle school play and invited me to play Jo March, the tomboy role. I read Louisa May Alcott and loved *Little Women* because it was about courtship, marriage, illness, and death in ordinary families like ours. After the drama coach introduced the play to the cast, she asked each character to memorize her part. I misunderstood and memorized the entire play instead of just my role. During rehearsals, I prompted the other actresses, which made me feel good to help. This mistake upset the coach, who phoned my mother and explained my error, claiming I was too intense about Jo March and assimilated her traits off and on stage. The drama coach informed Mother that when I played the tomboy off stage, I was destructive. For example, I removed a heavy cellar door leading from the stage to the school basement below it and removed bottles of Orange Crush to give to cast members. "Whose Orange Crush was it, anyway?" I wondered. The coach insisted to Mother that this was theft and not merely innocent climbing from one floor to another to quench our thirsts.

It surprised me that the coach also knew about my Saturday mischief and communicated the episode to Mother in detail. I hadn't yet had time to explain it to my mother myself. The coach inquired of Mother, "Can you imagine green grass sprinkled on your freshly varnished floors at home? Ask your tomboy daughter about it." As it happened, one Saturday afternoon, the school windows remained open to expel the odor from the newly varnished floors. The janitor not only left the windows open, but also neglected to collect the freshly cut green grass left in plastic bags near the open school window. These combined fragrances inspired me to sprinkle what I called "green coconut on chocolate frosting." To the coach and Mother, I tried to explain, "I did it because the green looked pretty on the brown floor, and it smelled good." Neither accepted the explanation. Mother insisted that I clean the mess and pay for the damages. The drama coach ended my acting career. I didn't understand why neither of them could empathize with me.

To remain a part of the theater, I often sat in the auditorium watching the rehearsal for a new play that was being cast. I felt alone and isolated as other pupils rehearsed their roles in new plays. I was convinced that I could play certain roles better and sat in the darkened theater wondering how to be cast in one of those roles.

During these middle school years, I preferred school to home because school had more resources. At home, we only had a few serious books—*Time Line of History*, *Five Major Religions*, The Bible, a dictionary, and classic English and American novels. We had even fewer magazines. The radio news was frequently filled with static whether the sound emanated from the small plastic green radio sitting on the kitchen cupboard or from the large varnished console radio in the living room. Few families owned televisions, and we were not among them. *The New York Times* was delivered only on Sundays, and all other days we received the slim daily city newspaper. Father read both papers before we were allowed to do so and he carried on a monologue without permitting us to talk.

In school, the pupils and teachers talked about ideas, and I could ask questions, which would be answered. School had its downside, though. Throughout the middle school years, my schoolmates were preoccupied with activities that held little interest for me until later years. They were occupied with gossip about the opposite sex, clothes, makeup, socializing, making and spending money, clothing and fads, and occasionally boys' sports. I was a good athlete and flattered by the invitations to play touch football with the boys. However, I often rejected their offers in order to satisfy my responsibilities to study, babysit, home chores, and performing tasks for others.

Doing tasks for others often involved me in accidents, which Mother rejected even more than illness. In the early grades, I think I was accident-prone, and Mother wanted no part of it. She was Freudian and believed accidents could be avoided. I thought Freud and Mother were wrong, but I had to make camouflages to avoid confrontations with Mother over accidents. For example, one freezing winter day, a good deed turned into a bad event. I offered to go to the store to buy a quart of milk for the elderly couple that lived across the street from us. It gave me the opportunity to raise money for my tree of life, and I also liked to do little chores for people. I went to the neighbor's house to pick up the empty glass milk bottle and coins for the purchase.

Enjoying running even though it was forbidden, I slipped on the icy sidewalk in front of the small, dilapidated church on the corner near our house and broke the bottle. The milk bottle cut my right hand, but I walked into the church to see if I could talk God into intervening in my mishap. I didn't believe in God, but He answered my prayers in the sunflower play, so maybe He would do it again.

The red, green, and blue vigil lights flickering in front of the Virgin Mary altar lured me in, and I begged the Virgin Mary to stop the bleeding as I knelt in front of her altar, praying for at least fifteen minutes. She did nothing, so I left the church and proceeded to the store where the owner and his wife gasped at the bleeding cut and the blood covering my winter jacket. It wasn't as bad as it looked, but they immediately drove me to my doctor who put in eleven stitches and put a cast on my hand. The procedure hurt, but I said nothing. When the doctor finished,

I thanked him and asked that it be kept a secret from Mother. His only comment was, "So you're still playing cat and mouse with your mother. Time to stop, don't you think?" I disagreed, but said nothing. I hadn't yet devised a plan to hide my cast, so I pulled down my sweater sleeve to cover it. This was a difficult feat because of my unusually long arms. Mother must have observed the cast, but she did not acknowledge it. Since my right hand couldn't function, I began to write with my left hand and I remain mildly ambidextrous.

That same winter, still wearing my cast, I was playing on the slide on the school grounds. The cast was awkward and resulted in an inadequate grasp of the handles on the slide, causing me to fall off the top onto a piece of ice, which cut my forehead prominently. This time, Elvera walked me to my Aunt Esther's house across the alley from school, and she and Aunt Esther bandaged the wound instead of taking me to my doctor. The scar on my forehead did not readily heal, so they cut my hair into bangs to cover it. It was another camouflage that avoided Mother's agitation.

Academics Compete with Fashion: High School—1945–1953

At 3:30 every afternoon, my girlfriends met after classes at the drugstore across the street from our retail store, where I worked. I envied their social time and tried to figure how I might join them. For me, high school was occupied with study and work and not social time. The private high school I attended placed me in the gifted academic track, which automatically increased my study time. In that educational era, the teachers used tracking, which meant that if a student was placed in the A track for one course, the student was placed in the A track for all courses. Recently, a more enlightened approach has been to organize students homogeneously, which means that students are grouped by talent. An A student in chemistry doe not necessarily indicate an A student in a literature course. Tracking requires an increase in study time because not all students are good in all subjects. For instance, I was better in the humanities than in the sciences and therefore had to double my study time in the sciences to maintain a high average. I was dissatisfied with less than a 95% average so I dedicated many hours to studying to attain an A average in all subjects.

Additionally, the faculty appointed me the editor of the high school yearbook, which required a design for the yearbook, the collection of cameo photos of the faculty, staff, and students, action shots of all activities, and copy to report the year. My most demanding job was motivating other seniors to work with me in the early mornings before classes or on Saturdays. The schedule in past years was arranged for after school hours, but I had to work at the store then. Many seniors were unwilling to make the sacrifice, resulting in a minority of three or four students, usually from the visual arts. The result was greater editorial control by the few.

Traditionally, for at least twenty-five years, the yearbook design included a heavy, navy blue padded cover with the content organized chronologically. As editor, I chose an unconventional design, a thin scarlet cover with content organized thematically. Time was the symbol to divide the year, the seasons, the events, and overriding philosophical concepts. We designed the cover with bold black and white division pages with a large clock on each, specifying appropriate times for different themes —"time to work," time to play," "time to save your soul," "time to contribute," and so on. The small staff and I thought the book was stylish and smart, but when the student body received the yearbook at the end of the year, they rejected it.

As I walked into the classrooms to deliver the books, the students made snide remarks like "We should have expected Marie to design an unorthodox book, she always goes her own way." Some requested refunds. I felt the height of accomplishment and elation when the book came off the press, but it soon spiraled down to the nadir of despair. I learned to display no emotions because I knew the book was good, which was validated when the book received an award from all of the yearbook publishers for one of the outstanding yearbooks of 1953. I was usually a pacesetter. However, the students returned the next year to publish the traditional yearbook to which they had grown accustomed and attached.

Because I had to pay my own tuition and expenses at the private high school I attended, employment for me was essential. Fortunately, my brother-in-law, Linda's husband, offered me a position as a sales clerk at his women's specialty retail store, where he was manager. I worked after school hours, when classes were dismissed, some Saturdays, and at times late into the night when the store had additional jobs, like unpacking merchandise or attaching price tags. My brother-in-law hired me to sell fashion clothing about which I knew nothing because of lack of exposure. I owned no new outfits but wore my sisters' hand-me-downs. I had to be a fast study to keep the position. In one year, I learned merchandising and selling techniques, and after the initial year I was asked to dress the mannequins and decorate the large display windows. Imagination was my mentor; I transformed the traditional windows to new approaches for which I had no prototypes. I learned the field fast and by the third year of employment, the manager invited me to fly to New York with the store's sportswear buyer to purchase women's sportswear for the store. The buyer inquired about my parents' attitude toward their sixteen-year-old daughter traveling to New York unchaperoned. When I asked my parents, as I assumed, they hadn't given it a thought and they supported the travel and the new experience for me.

In the New York Garment District for several weeks each summer, I was given an informal extended course in women's retail. The experiences were not only about buying and selling but addressed style and treatment of buyers, finances and markdowns of merchandise. Markdowns were a serious topic because therein lay the profit. Fewer markdowns indicated better merchandise choices and increased the profit. In the women's retail business, a store had one chance a season to succeed. The market was fickle, and styles changed rapidly.

The manufacturers' showrooms in New York were small, shabby, hectic, and managed by experienced older Jewish men. Few women worked in the Garment District except as secretaries or assistants. These businessmen understood their market, and they worked the clock around in season. They had the capacity for total recall, keeping everything in their heads—what merchandise was in, what merchandise was out, what the style numbers were, what the costs and discounts of all items were, the purchases buyers made from year to year, the dates of purchases. These wholesalers welcomed me to work in their shops and often invited me to model their new sportswear styles. My reward was a gift of the styles that they believed would not sell. They discarded many attractive expensive suits because their "shelf life" would be too long and they would end up on sale. I was a grateful recipient of the suits, excited to wear such high fashions and new designs.

Liking all manners of celebration, I especially appreciated the ritual for closing a deal between seller and buyer. When a sale, varying from as little as $10,000 to as much as $100,000 or more, was consummated, the seller offered the buyer a shot glass filled with warm scotch and no ice. Both drank the shot in one gulp. I thought the taste must be repugnant and hoped that I would not have to participate. I did think the ritual a good closure and preferable to a glass of champagne. Only once several years later, did I again see warm scotch drunk this way, and that was by my Jewish father-in-law before dinner.

I implemented a number of habits from the New York market when I returned to the store, and I also incorporated them into my academic studies and general approach to life. Taking their lead, I learned to store data to memory, organize concepts, outline the major points of a merchandise order, and add relevant details. I arranged all of this information in notebooks by year. Notebooks became my hallmark, and to this day, I continue to use this organization technique for most tasks, now owning more than 300 notebooks, used for at least sixty projects varying from teaching to fundraising.

Advanced employment at the store included more interesting positions. I learned about fashion and taught customers to break their former habits of dress and clothe themselves in different and newer styles. It pleased many women to alter their appearances, and it pleased me to be successful.

I was salaried by commission, which was lucrative. I learned the women's retail field rapidly and seriously considered rejecting college and making a career of women's fashion. I developed a flair and liking for fashion. The salary doubled a starting teacher's salary and the field was far more glamorous. However, my brother-in-law insisted on the value of a college education, and I accepted his advice, reflecting my oldest sister's regret that she had not earned a college degree.

Numerous diverse and intense responsibilities—studying for A-track courses, selling clothing after school, traveling to New York to buy sportswear, editing a yearbook—did not interfere with my graduating in the top ten of my high school class of 300 students. I enjoyed using some of my graduation gift money to buy the remaining foreign babies to paste on my "tree of life."

Money Determines College Choice—1953–1957

The decision to attend college was solely mine, but I did receive a little persuasion from my brother-in-law, Robert. No member of my family completed a four-year college degree before I attended, so no one offered advice except the command, "Go." Our high school did not employ a college counselor on campus to discuss career goals, so no one was available to discuss college choices or to introduce available government grants provided for bright students with insufficient funds. Like high school, I was accountable for financing college on my own.

Ambitious, eager, and determined, as well as unprepared, uninformed, and doubtful, my college education was fragmentary at best.

Lack of college information, inadequate funds, and a poor geographic location were variables that determined my college choice, which turned out to be a bad fit for me. When I was ready to attend college in 1953, there were two colleges in my vicinity. I chose the University of Minnesota–Minneapolis because it offered low tuition and was near my home, where there was available public transportation. I didn't own a car.

As a college freshman, to my surprise and disappointment, I realized the curriculum was only slightly less difficult than in the secondary school's track for the gifted student. There were exceptions, especially in the sciences, in which I gained a great interest.

The wealth from Minnesota's iron ore industry financed The Rangers, a group of students from Northern Minnesota who were invited to share in the largess of Minnesota's natural resource—iron ore—and attend college tuition-free. The Rangers were a group of Serbian males, dark and attractive, whose families were the original settlers of the iron mining fields. They were a fun-loving and athletic group who were disinclined to study. They set the ethos of the college, and I complained about their value system to the dean. Furthermore, I made it a point not to date a Ranger. They had poor study habits, which lowered the grade curve. Their drinking habits had a negative effect on the social life of the school. I organized a group of colleagues to talk with the dean about the negative effect the Rangers were perpetrating at the university.

The dean agreed with our interpretation, but was unable to change the course of events.

I had difficulty finding my academic focus the first quarter of college, which caused me to lose myself intellectually. It was the first time I earned only average grades and did not excel, which was unacceptable to me. Unclear of purpose, unmotivated by the college atmosphere, and over committed to my part-time women's retail job, I realized I made the wrong college choice both intellectually and socially. I raised my freshman average and completed the freshman year in order to transfer from the state university to a private girls' college.

I used my entire college savings to finance my sophomore and junior years so I could attend a college twenty miles outside St. Cloud. I had to consider how to finance my senior year, but postponed that decision for a later day.

Old red brick federal buildings constituted the girls' university located in the country. The campus was accessible by public, college, and private transportation. I enrolled as a day student, but arranged to use a room in the dormitory when one was vacant. The university permitted me to live as a part-time resident student in exchange for doing clerical work. College was an exceptional pleasure as a resident because of the access to the library and the other college resources, which could be used during the large blocks of study time. The university emphasized scholarship, conveyed an ambience of propriety, and demanded lady-like deportment. We were required to wear hats to and from campus. For lunch, we dined in the lunchroom. Lunch was served formally for all students at noon on tables covered with white linen tablecloths complemented by white linen napkins and name rings that specified the seating arrangement. Each student was assigned to a table headed by a professor, who identified those students lacking correct table manners. Some classes were held later in the day for the purpose of teaching good table manners. Given my family background, I knew I would not have to attend those classes.

Academic classes were small with reading and writing as the prime teaching methods. The workload was heavy, and the professors were demanding, but effective. The atmosphere was conducive to learning. I chose sociology as my major field because the chairman was outstanding, and the field gave a general introduction to ideas for someone unsure of her career—like me. The school offered a credible modern dance program in which I participated in a limited way due to lack of time. The college was a big promoter of the arts, and the professors arranged art exhibitions, dramas, and concerts.

When living at home, in order to maintain a high grade average, I awakened at four o'clock every morning to study when the house was quiet. First, I had to adjust the heat because the Minnesota chill caused a cold house in the early mornings during at least three school quarters. In the quiet, cool, and dark house, I sat at the dining room table and studied for at least two hours until I took the seven o'clock bus to the college. Balancing retail work and college studies became increasingly difficult, but I had little choice because I was already in debt.

Several times, the retail store had to send a driver to campus so I could complete sales orders. Mr. Silverman, a jewelry salesman, came frequently. He was from out of the city and arrived in a huge, ostentatious black Cadillac, which embarrassed me in front of the other students who teased me about dating older Jewish salesmen. I was grateful for the store's willingness to let me continue my job, which was now a necessity, and I continued to work at the retail store. It is true that I preferred Jewish men with whom I became familiar in the garment district in New York.

An all male university was located five miles from the girls' university. I dated conventionally and did not search for what the co-eds deemed "a good catch"—a man who offered a glamorous life secured by money. I didn't have much time for social life, but if desired, the opposite sex was available. The university for men enrolled a ratio of six males to one female. Located between the two universities were dives—places where students congregated to drink beer, dance, meet the opposite sex, and socialize. I spent a few evenings socializing at the dives with a group of colleagues, swapping stories about the week, dancing when invited, and drinking Cokes in preference to alcoholic beverages. When transportation was available, a group of girls and I drove into the city to attend concerts, the theater, or movies.

As time passed, my interest in the business world began to diminish and my interest in the humanities bloomed. The demands of scholarship, the retail business, the clerical hours worked at school, and socialization exhausted me, and I worked intensively, going to bed late, getting up early, and skipping meals when necessary. I bordered on making myself sick. I had to study and work without a break or a vacation for eight years—four years of high school and four years of college—to meet my goals. As college graduation neared, I had to push forward harder and faster with a debt owed the college and no teaching position secured for that fall.

For me, college graduation was traumatic and not a joyous event. I received the award for the outstanding student in sociology, but my diploma and the award were withheld due to unpaid tuition. I couldn't ask my parents to pay final costs because of their limited funds.

After the graduation ceremony, I visited the college dean and convinced her that I would complete the tuition payment in August, but the dean did not release the diploma or the award until tuitions were paid.

My parents never visited the campus throughout my three years in attendance. The graduation ceremony brought them to the university for the first time. Following the ceremony, I abandoned my parents instead of showing them around campus. I also escaped the crowds and festivities and hid in the library, weeping hysterically. Unsure of the reason for the tears, I felt on the verge of a breakdown. Maybe college graduation is similar to postpartum blues that mothers experience after the birth of a child. I was now detached from the university and without a new destination. I was a displaced person.

Wishing to congratulate me on the Sociology Award, my sociology professor found me in the library. But when she discovered me, I burst out in tears. She tried to soothe me, but I couldn't tell her what was wrong because I didn't know. Embarrassed, I assured her that I was crying from happiness. It was in fact despair. I wiped my eyes with a Kleenex and searched for my parents, whom I blamed for my ordinary education. In retrospect, it seemed like a wasted four years of college. I was much more capable and qualified intellectually, but it was the lack of economic resources that prohibited me from attending an Eastern college like the heavenly seven, Princeton, or one of the other prestigious schools. I realized that geography and economics were big impediments for college. I could not understand why my friends had the financial resources, but no desire to set their college goals higher. They were happy to enroll in the college their parents and siblings attended.

In silence, my parents and I drove home together. I made them sad, and it should have been a happy occasion. They were first generation immigrants and their daughter graduated from college with honors. Neither spoke a word. We pulled into the driveway, and when we entered the house, ironically, on the kitchen table stood at least a dozen vases filled with red roses, yellow tulips, purple lilacs, orange tiger lilies, white orchids, and other flowers. With disinterest, I read the congratulatory notes from my siblings, colleagues, friends, and some of the boys I had dated, so that I could write thank you notes. Angrily, I arranged the flowers in a large cardboard box, which I padded with folded newspaper to secure the bottom, and delivered the flowers to the little old dilapidated church where I had fallen with the milk bottle when I was ten.

My graduation present in 1957 was Hodgkin's Disease. I struggled with three years of treatment for Hodgkin's Disease, and I completed two years of graduate school at the University of Minnesota, earning my master's degree in English.

At age twenty-six, in 1961, I married Nelson Stone, a surgeon I had met the previous year. After meeting at an open house, Nelson and I dated each other until the completion of his final year as a surgical resident at the

University of Minnesota. I taught at Alexander Ramsey High School, but my intention was to stop teaching and remain at home to raise a family. It was a turning point in each of our lives. Nelson completed his residency in surgery at Minnesota.

I had rejected an earlier proposal of marriage from another physician, but now the main question was no longer whether or not I should marry, but where I should get married. My mother was deceased, so I had no particular desire to be married in Minneapolis. Dr. Stone's parents strongly disapproved of our marriage because of my health status, which could not assure my bearing children. The problem stemmed from the fact that my husband's mother lost sixteen members of her family in the Holocaust, and she was determined to have grandchildren, which I could not promise. Nelson was adamant about his decision to marry me and told his mother she had to accept me or he would reject her for the remainder of our lives. She was on the edge of a breakdown, but she wasn't about to lose her only son, so she consented. To appease his mother, we were married in the reform temple by Rabbi Lelyveld in Cleveland, Ohio, my husband's birthplace.

The day I arrived in Cleveland, I wanted to return to Minneapolis immediately. I was fearful of another health-related rejection and I did not feel welcome at the Stone house. The maid of honor, my oldest sister, and the best man, her husband, were in Cleveland for the nuptials and insisted, "You went this far in this relationship and we won't let you stop now." They persuaded me to marry Dr. Stone despite my reservations. Neither knew all the problems plaguing me, but if not for their advice, I would have returned to Minneapolis a single woman.

After the marriage, my husband and I returned to Minneapolis for a brief period to finalize his general surgical specialty and his Doctor of Philosophy degree at the University of Minnesota. We then moved to Chicago where he was invited to co-head and develop a burn unit. Eventually, he planned to complete residencies in hand and in plastic and reconstructive surgery at Northwestern University. These specialties were strengths at Northwestern Medical School.

In Chicago, other opportunities arose—performing the earliest change of sex surgeries with Dr. Stutteville and introducing laser surgery before other surgeons did. A serious student with a doctorate and four surgical specialties, a lover of classical music with a perfect ear, a photographer of flowers, a collector of relic medicine bottles, and a writer of medical articles and books, Dr. Stone was happy to live in Chicago with its superb exposure to the medical specialties in which he was interested in and the arts of which he was a great connoisseur.

I disliked giving up my position at Alexander Ramsey High School, which Superintendent Williams saved for me, but women had little choice in the sixties except to follow the career paths of their husband. In Chicago for the next five years, Nelson studied while I taught.

Chapter Six:

Radiation Causes Reproductive Problems

In the mid-seventies, we still had not conceived a child. It seemed to me that the odds favoring conception were diminishing. Radiation treatments were possible causes of sterility, but I felt sure of winning my battle with health. I was shocked that my bi-annual checkup revealed that I had reproductive problems. Several times I was hospitalized for dilatation and curettage, popularly known as a "DC," a minor surgical procedure in which the gynecologist scrapes the lining of the uterus to check for irregularities. During this procedure, my physician diagnosed endometriosis, an illness that further interferes with childbearing. The gynecologist also diagnosed cervical cancer, a cancer with few ramifications. These reproductive problems caused pain and some caused sterility, but they were not chronic and after successful surgeries, I felt well. All I had to show for the reproductive problems, however, was what the gynecologist jokingly called a bikini scar.

Description of Endometriosis

Endometriosis is a benign disorder characterized by the presence and proliferation of endometrial tissue outside of the endometrial cavity. Endometriosis afflicts eight to ten percent of women of childbearing age, usually between ages thirty to forty. The primary symptom is pain, and many women suffer from pain in the pelvic area. Pain is usually in the form of excessive cramping during menstrual periods or during or after intercourse. The fertility rate is significantly reduced and fifty to sixty percent of women with endometriosis become infertile. The diagnosis can be confirmed by direct visualization usually through a laparoscope tube. Other procedures include ultrasound scans, barium enemas with x-ray, computed tomography (CT), and magnetic resonance imaging (MRI). Their usefulness in diagnosis is limited.[3]

Description of Cervical Cancer

Cervical Cancer, in my case cancer in situ, the first stage, was diagnosed.

"The cervix is the lower end of the uterus, which extends into the vagina. Of cancers of the female reproductive system, cervical cancer is the second most common in all women and the most common in younger women. It usually affects women between the ages of thirty-five and fifty-five . . . Risk for cervical cancer seems to increase as the number of sexual partners increases . . . About eighty-five

---

[3] Information taken from the *Merck Manual of Medical Information*, 1997, pp. 1194–95.

percent of cervical cancers are squamous cell carcinomas . . . Cervical cancer can penetrate deep beneath the surface of the cervix, enter the lymphatic vessels that line the inside of the cervix and then spread to other parts of the body . . . The Pap test can accurately and inexpensively detect up to ninety percent of cervical cancers . . ."[4]

Description of Hysterectomy

A hysterectomy is a surgical procedure to remove a woman's entire womb, as well as all of the tissues holding the womb in place, the top of the vagina, and all of the lymph nodes around the womb.

I struggled for most of the late seventies with reproductive disorders that interfered with my getting pregnant, but then my gynecologist told me I needed a hysterectomy. Now a different set of destructive forces plagued me. In the sixties, I was physically distressed, but now I became emotionally distressed. I was ten years older, married, without a child, and my life seemed out of my control.

The year following the hysterectomy, my husband and I discussed adoption, but he was opposed to the idea. Age was looming as a significant barrier for adoption. We were thirty-five and forty years old respectively that August and September.

The hysterectomy was defeating, but I couldn't give in. I was sure my husband would help me and his love would strengthen me. After ten days in the hospital following the hysterectomy, Nelson picked me up on Sunday morning

---

[4] *Merck Manual of Medical Information*, 1997, pp. 1212–13.

and filled the backseat of his new brown Jaguar with the beautiful bouquets of flowers sent to me by my friends. We hugged each other mightily and drove home. His presence, the smell of his new car, and the bouquets of fall flowers were all illuminated by the glorious fall sunlight, which encouraged me to believe that we could re-define our lives with or without children. We parked the car in our garage and Nelson carried the flowers upstairs to our apartment.

Nelson left for a medical conference in San Francisco. After he left, the house was deadly quiet. The flowers couldn't fill the emptiness. I telephoned my friend, the late Golda Sher, and asked her to visit me. She and her husband, Maurie, altered their Sunday afternoon plans and joined me for tea.

I couldn't give Nelson the child he wanted and felt guilty. What could I give him? In the 1970s, adoption was a more difficult process than in 2000. The couple had to have good physical and economic credentials and illustrate that they could care for the child. It helped to know a professional in the field, who would provide a good reference. Adoption of infants from other countries was not on the radar screen for another ten years. I intended to adopt a child on my own, believing that my husband would learn to love that child. Adoption by one member of a couple, however, especially one with a potentially terminal illness, was impossible, no matter the effort extended.

Childless Marriage Unsatisfactory

I experienced a period of good health with the exception of short episodes of treatment for Hodgkin's Disease.

After we married, we lived in Chicago in a large, white

contemporary house on top of a hill. It was not an ostentatious house, but it did have colonnades. It had a chair-like swing on the open porch that held three people. There I sat swinging or writing, stimulated by the flower garden planted with pink and blue pansies, yellow gladiolas, white flocks, purple lilacs, and jewel colored asters. Tall evergreen trees surrounded the periphery of the grounds providing the privacy I sought.

I awaited the birth of a daughter, who was to be named Alexandra because I liked the androgyny of the nickname, Alex, and symbolically Alexandra began and ended with an A, a symbol I invented for the Stone children. Alex only lived in my dream. At age four, I dressed her in crisp white cotton pinafores, braided her golden hair, and walked hand in hand with her to school every day. If I could not have a child, I would teach hundreds of students. I would begin by teaching at a suburban school, then a girl's school, and when Alex attended private school full time, I would teach part-time at the same school, scheduling my day so it was compatible with Alex's.

I often spent late summer and fall afternoons composing fantasies in solitude. One was that, as an author of prize-winning articles and books, combined with a teaching salary and investments, I amassed sufficient wealth to establish a private foundation, which I designated to finance the education of poor children. The community's recognition of my altruism would motivate invitations to a variety of boards: Urban Gateways, Big Brothers and Sisters, the Children's Zoo Playground, the Saint Joseph Hospital, and others. I would be invited to become head of several fundraising projects, to chair social balls, provide leadership for re-building a children's playground, create a bowl-a-thon, and other events. My tastes for volunteering were catholic, but always child-centered.

In the beginning of our marriage, I occupied my time renting and decorating an apartment on Chicago's north side where I wanted the daughter of my dream to attend one of several excellent private schools. After I completed decorating a two-bedroom apartment, I began to search for other tasks to occupy my time.

Worse Things Can Happen in Marriage Besides Death

I had to agree with Dr. Mosser, who asserted earlier, "Worse things can happen in marriage besides death." This moment seemed the nadir. When my husband returned from San Francisco, he professed to having a good time listening to effective papers well delivered by his colleagues and by renowned professors. Sailing beyond the Golden Gate Bridge was a dramatic experience for him, even if it was very cold. I felt my envy rise. Before this, I had always traveled with Nelson whether it was for delivering a lecture in Prague or attending a meeting in New York. As I helped him unpack his clothing, my envy diminished. For me, sex was allied with having him. Nelson and I had contrary goals. Medicine had not yet advanced the new fertility theories that became popular in the nineties.

That fall, several events collided and changed our lives dramatically. Dr. Stone's father died unexpectedly from an aortic aneurysm. We immediately drove to Cleveland to sit Shiva and to arrange for Nelson's family funeral. Driving the several hundred miles from Chicago to Cleveland, I had this eerie feeling that Nelson's father's estate would exclude his son because of the lack of an offspring, and it would name his mother and sister as beneficiaries. I suggested this to Nelson, wanting to prepare him for the possibility. When I shared my thoughts, he called it absurd and foolish, saying, "Such an act is unheard of between a Jewish father and his son."

Upon our arrival in Cleveland, Dr. Stone's mother felt horrified to deliver to her son the news that he had been excluded from the family will. She loved him dearly and money was not the issue, but the absence of any explanation from his father was devastating.

Nelson's elderly mother would be living alone, so we welcomed her to live with us, but she had other plans.

Nelson was experiencing his change of life crisis. He keenly felt the rejection by his father, which stimulated his anger and caused his sadness. I remembered how Hodgkin's Disease had caused a friend of mine to break up a much less serious relationship.

Sundays became the worst days of the week. I didn't want us to remain home, so I focused on motivating Nelson to do something. At times, we visited his aunt and uncle in the suburbs where we spent parts of the afternoon walking through the woods, playing tennis on the public courts near his uncle's house, or watching a sports event on television. Previous infrequent television watchers, we became curious about a new show on television called *Columbo*. These activities enlivened Nelson, but he often retired to his uncle's library by mid-afternoon, turned off the lights, and fell asleep. He would awaken for dinner, which we all joined in cooking. Occasionally, he would join us for a picnic supper at a Ravinia concert, which was within walking distance of his uncle's house. Sundays took a colossal effort to design.

Rejection was excruciating. Each evening over the next months I lay in bed and watched the shadows on the ceiling. It was difficult to recover emotionally from the female problems under these circumstances. I wasn't even sure I wanted to recover. I had been working diligently to overcome Hodgkin's Disease and making good strides. To give in now seemed foolish, but I had to learn to manage several illnesses—Hodgkin's Disease, cervical cancer in situ, endometriosis, and a hysterectomy.

The combination of Hodgkin's Disease, multiple surgeries on my reproductive system, and infertility ruined our marriage, which led to our separation in 1978 and subsequent divorce. Nelson and I remained friendly, and in times of crisis, I called upon him to help me, which he willingly did. Five years later, he remarried, and his wife bore him two daughters. Concurrently, I earned a doctorate degree and became the other Dr. Stone.

Chapter Seven:

Teaching Motivates

Teaching at a Catholic Girls' School—1968

Waiting for my husband to arrive home one Friday evening to take me out to dinner, I stood gazing from the large bedroom window, watching the red tail lights of the cars form a beaded chain on Lake Shore Drive for four blocks northward from our apartment. There, I identified Immaculata, a small Catholic girls' school.

The following Monday, I decided to inquire if the school could use a teacher. I phoned the school, explaining, "I'm a Jew and not Catholic, but I am a good teacher who will work without remuneration." I realized that Catholic schools suffered from tight budgets, but I was doubtful about its response because I didn't think Immaculata would accept a non-Catholic on its staff in the 1960s.

The school year had already begun, but with great enthusiasm, Sister Margaret Mary, the principal, asked me if I could visit the next day and spend some time interviewing with the administrators and the faculty. On Tuesday, I arrived at the convent and an English teacher met me and ushered me into the senior literature class. She introduced me to the girls and asked if I could teach Flannery O'Connor, a Catholic author who wrote *The Violent Shall Bear It Away* and whom the girls were studying with their previous teacher. I guess O'Connor was to be my test. I assured her that I could, and she put me to the task. She left the classroom and I began class at once, knowing the American classic well. Dead silence prevailed for the first several minutes until I inquired, "What is the silence about?" The girls responded in unison that they could not sit down and begin class until I sat. I could not learn to begin class by sitting down, but the class and I made an arrangement. The girls would say their opening prayer to which they would add, "Be seated, Mrs. Stone."

Following my trial day, I was invited to teach the senior literature class for the remainder of the year. The girls had been trained in textual analysis and most liked to read fiction. Their first love, however, was to divert from the text and talk about life. I wanted to achieve that goal for them because a key variable in learning is to begin with the child's interest. My plan was to divide the text into literary elements—the narrative, the characters, the structure, the symbols, and the dominant themes, after which I asked three different seniors to choose and explain one element aloud for the class and to interrelate the element to some aspect of their family, friends, or their lives. The class wrote a cumulative list on the chalkboard of the aspects in life that the elements of the novel evoked and then wrote vignettes about selected titles, which we read aloud in class. Engaged in the lesson, the 8:30 class began earlier because students arrived in the room before class was scheduled. The method was a successful way to teach literature, to teach life, and to improve students' speaking and writing skills.

At Christmas time, the nuns invited my husband and me for the Christmas celebration dinner, and the principal asked me at that time if I would instruct the young novitiates to teach literature. I consulted with my husband, who reflected, "If you do get pregnant, you could still complete next year." I informed the principal that I would teach the young nuns until the end of the year.

Secure, joyful, active and fun-loving characterized my husband's and my relationship during the first decade of our marriage. Others considered us the model couple and we became the envy of our friends and colleagues. We bought a large apartment in a vintage building with expansive windows overlooking the children's playground, the zoo, Lincoln Park, and Lake Michigan. It was the perfect place for our anticipated daughter, Alexandra, to play. Several private schools were within walking distance, and in the rear of the apartment, we planned to build a nursery. A large dining room permitted us to entertain friends and to arrange parties for fundraising, which was my long-range commitment. I was invited to become a member of the hospital board, accepted the appointment, and made it my goal to raise one million dollars for St. Joseph Hospital in gratitude for winning my battle with Hodgkin's Disease. It took a group of us about ten years, but we succeeded in achieving the goal.

Photos of us filled the northside newspapers, which served the neighborhood where we lived. Diverse activities crowded our lives, and Nelson and I enjoyed many interests in common. We studied and wrote together, attended the Chicago symphony on Friday nights during the season, and visited and collected art at the numerous Chicago galleries. We owned tickets for the opening nights of several theaters ranging from the Goodman to the Steppenwolf. Some nights we went to the movies, for which we had a passion. We also often attended auctions and purchased oriental sculptures, furniture, and figurines to complete the decoration of our recently renovated 1920s apartment. The forty-foot gallery was the ideal showcase to display these art objects. We took pleasure in using the apartment for fundraising events, which ranged from brunches for the hospital to cocktail parties for neighbors to ask them to join in building a playground.

Arranging a Stone Salon—1980

Again, teaching became my survival. I taught private school students and undergraduates. In 1969, I was invited to team-teach junior and senior English and literature with Dr. Thomas, the principal of the Francis W. Parker Independent School. Dr. Thomas lived in the same building as did I, and he invited me to join the staff of the Parker School despite my illness. After a year of satisfactory work with Dr. Thomas, he advanced me to chairman of the English Department. Professionally, I ascended the ladder of increasing responsibility as I was subsequently appointed the first dean of students, then the first college counselor for women, and finally the dean of curriculum. One more step to go. The top step was the headmistress, but with my health record, the top position, while tempting, was unthinkable because I could not promise the stability that would be required for a school.

Each position required greater influence on the school. Except for dean of studies, the other positions are self-explanatory. The dean of studies shaped, implemented, and oversaw the course of study for grades 6–12. My approach was experimental and collaborative. The faculty experimented with transforming the schedule and all the courses for high school students. Several courses were designed to be interdisciplinary in nature like combining English and history—"The Victorian English Writers and the Influence of Europe on Their Writing." Other courses combined science and literature—"The Life and Works of Galileo Galilei." Still, others were new in content and approach like "Health and Physical Education," "Religion and Literature, and Community Service." The materials for each course filled notebooks that constituted the first curriculum library.

I combined teaching classes as I headed curriculum, finding the greatest pleasure in coming to know the members of the senior class. To familiarize the students with each other and with me, each year I invited two groups of twenty-five seniors to my home to what I labeled the "Stone Salon," imitating Gertrude Stein's French seminars. All students met in my large living room, and one individual student or a panel of students presented ideas on a novel or novels we studied in class. Mostly, the class analyzed the novels in a most sophisticated manner. We tried different techniques.

Following the salon, we adjourned to the dining room for a small repast. That format permitted me to communicate with mature intellects and students of character. For example, one junior became acquainted with the African-American novel and invited novelist Rosemary Bray, age seventy-nine, a Parker published author, to present an analysis of her writing. The junior boy remained interested in writing, but when he attended Northwestern University, he had to switch majors to business because he had to earn tuition. Students represented a variety of economic levels. One male was born in the Cabrini Greene Projects, where money was scarce. One intellectually capable male was wealthy and excelled at Harvard Medical School. He assisted with Habitat for Humanity and other valuable social service organizations.

In a new writing class, which I developed, history was kept alive. Students helped me to write *Between Home and Community* (1975) to celebrate the seventy-fifth anniversary of the school. Others helped me to write and stage a narrative on the life of Colonel Francis Wayland Parker, the school's founder. Students researched background materials for *The Progressive Legacy* (2001), the hundredth anniversary text.

Today, many students communicate with me, informing me that at least one-third of them are professional writers, including the renowned Jonathan Alter, who writes for *Newsweek*, David Dunlap, David Stenn, Rosemary Bray, and several other recognized national authors. Parker School was also known for several well-known actresses like Anne Heche, Daryll Hannah, Lisa Hanh, and others. It is exactly the kind of school I would have wished for my child, Alex, to attend.

Teaching writing made me an accomplished author as it did the students. Because of my stroke, I had to learn to type with one hand, but I wouldn't give in, and wrote to publish *The Progressive Legacy*, and presently, I am writing my memoirs.

Chapter Eight:
A Geographic Move

A Hint of Business—1981

I now had choices at school—I could take a sabbatical leave after teaching for fifteen years between 1969 and 1983 and travel more; I could teach at the university; or I could address another long-term goal and invest in a startup company. I chose to further my interest in business. The roots stemmed from working in women's retail while in high school. I established two goals: I would travel, since I was feeling well, and I would invest in a startup company. I traveled to France and concluded the first part of my vacation in the French Riviera. From there, I flew to Israel where I was invited to present a paper, "Education for the Gifted." On my return flight from Israel, I met Mr. Anthony Evans, a former soccer player and businessman from England and South Africa. Mr. Evans discovered that I was intrigued by distance learning, especially the use of print and electronic media for teaching at distant sites— which turned out to be the major content involved in his new company.

Mr. Evans's new company in San Diego primarily manufactured down converters—converters that transmitted limited programs and excluded others. For example, American television could be excluded by Saudi Arabia and other Middle Eastern countries, which was their wish. In 1989, the plan was that Arabsat, the satellite for Arabian countries, would be constructed. Mr. Evans had not yet moved to San Diego with his wife and two sons, and had a great deal of work to do to develop his company. At this point, 1981, I joined the company. I hired the CEO, consulted with lawyers, and asked my friend, a realtor from Houston, to chair the board of trustees.

Several years later as the company began to grow, the CEO invited six investors from Greece, who offered to purchase the company. I was furious at first because I had just built the company and now it was on the market. However, when I discussed the transaction with my lawyers, they were enthusiastic about the purchase asserting, "You developed the company to sell it and make money, right?" "I suppose I did," I responded. Mr. Evans and I sold the company and indeed made a handsome profit.

While living in San Diego, a friend of mine formerly from Minneapolis, Joan Bernstein, introduced me to her friend, a physician. I told Joan that I would be interested in meeting him, but only for a glass of wine as a friend, nothing more, because I had been seriously dating Dr. Alvin Tarlov for the past ten years. Dr. Tarlov lived and worked in several different parts of the country during the twenty-five years of our acquaintainship. He was chairman of the department of internal medicine when at the University of Chicago, then he headed the Henry J. Kaiser

Foundation and moved to San Francisco. After eight years, he became a professor at the Harvard School of Public Health and returned to Boston. As he transferred, I could neither sustain a teaching position in the same city for an extended period of time, nor obtain new teaching positions easily with my poor health credentials.

I spent the summers and my vacation periods from school in LaJolla while I managed the business. After Mr. Evans and I sold the company, I rented university housing, which was more economical than a motel. I spent three-quarters of the year enjoying the ambience of LaJolla, but maintained my large apartment overlooking Lake Michigan in Chicago, where I spent the remaining months.

While in LaJolla, I experienced healthy years at first. I then began to have breathing problems and had a general checkup. I made an appointment with a pulmonologist. The pulmonologist sent me to a cardiologist for an angiogram. Ironically, the cardiologist then sent me to a thyroid specialist to consider a thyroidechtomy. The decision making process was confusing like a catch-22, so I returned to the University of Chicago Hospital to clarify the ambiguity. There, I was diagnosed with thyroid cancer. I proceeded to have a thyroidectomy by a world renowned endocrine surgeon, Dr. Edwin Kaplan.

Thyroid Surgery is Seamless

"Thyroid cancer is more common in people who have been treated with radiation to the head, neck, or chest . . . Most thyroid nodules are not cancerous and thyroid cancers can generally be cured . . . A painless lump in the neck is usually the first sign of thyroid cancer. When doctors find a nodule in the thyroid gland, they request several tests. A thyroid scan determines whether the nodule is functioning . . . a fine needle biopsy for examination under the microscope . . . the best way to determine whether the nodule is cancerous."[5]

In Chicago, the thyroidectomy went smoothly. It was neither a difficult disease nor a difficult surgery. When I awakened from surgery, I was surprised to be greeted by a resident doctor, who was a former student of mine. That was the good news; the bad news was that I had the potential of losing my voice, which would present a problem for teaching. Still a naive patient, I was mistakenly offered a call button for self-administering morphine, which I used often. It felt good, but I took too much. I was delirious before a medical person arrived. The thyroid cancer caused few long-range problems except the lack of easeful and effective swallowing.

[5] *Merck Manual of Medical Information*, 1997, p. 780.

Chapter Nine:

Poor Health Abounds

Breast Cancer—A Surprise

Following through with my general checkup, my cardiologist examined my breasts. That November, I had a mammogram and received a clean bill of health, so I disagreed with my doctor when he said I had a lump in my breast. But I took his advice and walked up to the eleventh floor to see a general surgeon, Dr. Wilson Hartz. My sister's death, which was caused by breast cancer, made me pessimistic. Dr. Hartz biopsied a spot on my left breast and the test confirmed breast cancer. He advised that I have a total mastectomy. Lumpectomies were unpopular at that time.

Description of Breast Cancer

"Breast cancer is classified by the kind of tissue in which it starts and by the extent of its spread. Cancer may start in the milk glands, milk ducts, fatty tissue, or connective tissue. Different types of breast cancers progress differently. Generalizations about particular types are based on similarities and how they're discovered, how they progress, and how they're treated. Some grow very slowly and spread to other parts of the body (metastasize) only after they become very large. Others are more aggressive, growing and spreading quickly. However, the same type of cancer may progress differently in different women . . . In situ cancer . . . is an early cancer that hasn't invaded or spread beyond its point of origin. In situ carcinoma accounts for more than fifteen percent of all breast cancers diagnosed in the United States. About ninety percent of all breast cancers start in the milk ducts or milk glands."[6]

Breast cancer changed the course of events that winter. I had planned a ski trip to plunge into the white powder of the manicured hills of Snowmass, Colorado. I enjoyed three marvelous skiing days, but on the third day I left the group to return to Chicago to keep my appointment with Dr. Hartz for breast surgery

At five o'clock on a cold, dark morning I arose to take a cab to the airport to embark on a flight to Chicago. I arrived at the O'Hare Airport, took a Boston Coach that I had previously ordered, dropped my luggage off at home, and proceeded to Northwestern University Hospital for breast surgery.

Alone, again, I went to the hospital where I remained for five days. I was then transferred to Rush Presbyterian Hospital for thirteen days of chemotherapy.

---

[6] *Merck Manual of Medical Information*, 1997, pp. 1198–99.

Description of Chemotherapy

"Although an ideal anticancer drug would destroy cancer cells without harming normal cells, no such drug exits. Despite the narrow margin between benefit and harm, however, many people with cancer can be treated with anticancer drugs (chemotherapy) and some can be cured. Today the side effects of chemotherapy can be minimized. Anticancer drugs are grouped into several categories: alkylating agents, antimetabolites, plant alkaloids, antitumor antibiotics, enzymes, hormones, and biologic response modifiers . . . combination chemotherapy is to use the drugs that work at different parts of the cells' metabolic processes, thereby increasing the likelihood that more cancer cells will be killed . . . the toxic side effects of chemotherapy may be reduced when drugs with different toxicities are combined, each at a lower dose than would be needed if one drug were used alone."[7]

I often hailed a cab to Rush Hospital, but some days my friend, Sallie Eley, or another friend's chauffeur drove me. They were most welcome because I worried that I might take ill in the cab. After arriving at the hospital, I took the elevator to the fifth floor where I saw my oncologist for a short while to discuss my health status based on the results of the chemotherapy. In the therapy room, I sat with needles in my wrists, which was debilitating. The other twenty patients' nausea exacerbated my own. I discovered that chewing ice alleviated some distress when taking chemotherapy, so I bought an ice machine for the cancer unit. Besides pain and nausea, all patients lost their

[7] *Merck Manual of Medical Information*, 1997, pp. 878–79.

hair. This time, I could offer advice about what kind of wigs to buy and where to purchase caps, scarves, and other paraphernalia for the head. The loss of hair three times in five years made me believe that my hair would not again reappear. However, it came in dark brown and curly.

After solving the hair problem, the next step was securing prostheses, which cost two hundred dollars on average. Finding prostheses for the breast was as difficult as finding wigs the first time. Access was available in catalogues, one specialty store in the city, and another store in the suburbs.

It was difficult to purchase and wear prostheses, but I soon learned to make the adjustment. Prostheses were heavy and seemed superfluous. Clothing and especially bathing suits are constructed to accommodate breast implants, which I didn't have.

To my surprise, I had to take physical therapy following breast cancer surgery to ward off stiffening of the left shoulder. Twice weekly, the therapist from Northwestern Hospital met with me in their therapy room in the basement of the hospital. I completed the regimen of therapy, but I later had to have treatments for lymphedema, swelling of the left arm, which is related to the surgery for breast cancer. After a while, chemotherapy did prove effective for me. I was able to return to teaching after a month.

Gall Bladder Attack Confused with Heart Attack

The Saturday night preceding open-heart surgery, I suffered from an excruciating pain, causing me to go to the emergency room at Northwestern University Hospital. It wasn't a heart attack as I expected, but a gall bladder attack, which necessitated immediate gall bladder surgery. I had been feeling well enough to order Dominick's Pizza. I had worked hard all week. I was anticipating a relaxing evening eating pizza and reading Nancy Milford's *Savage Beauty*, which my colleague, Bernard Kent Markwell sent to me, because the main female character reminded him of me. A half hour after the pizza arrived, my stomach started kicking and kicking harder. The pain was excruciating and became intolerable. I didn't want to go to the emergency room alone on a Saturday night, so I phoned my former husband and asked him to pick me up and take me. In thirty minutes, he was at my door. I spent the night at the ER to discover that the next morning Dr. Hartz would do gall bladder surgery.

I recovered within ten days from the surgery.

Description of Open-Heart Surgery with Two Valves Replaced

Standard open-heart surgery is performed on the heart while the bloodstream is diverted through a heart-lung machine. This surgery includes heart valve repairs or replacements, coronary artery bypass grafts, and repair of congenital abnormalities.

Following through with my general physical checkup, I continued with my Chicago cardiologist, Dr. Smith, because of shortness of breath, a complication that I gave too little attention. The cardiologist prescribed several diagnostic tests for my heart, but at that time did not indicate the need for any further medical attention. No family member joined me, so I was sure the doctor felt that he could not discuss the next step. Most doctors want patients to be joined by a family member when they are going to relate serious news.

I concluded with a final set of tests, which tired me. I went to the lobby to take a nap and accidentally fell sound asleep only to be awakened by the midnight janitor cleaning the floor. My purse and schoolbooks lay beside me and could have been stolen because I slept alone in the lobby.

On a cold winter evening after Christmas, Dr. Smith phoned to inform me that I required open-heart surgery. I didn't have the slightest idea of the nature of the surgical procedure. My cardiologist also informed me that he was retiring. I felt lost without Dr. Smith. He recommended that the surgery be done at the Mayo Clinic in Minnesota or at the Cleveland Clinic in Cleveland.

I checked out Minnesota, but the surgeon I wanted had become ill. I was pleased with what I had learned about the Cleveland Clinic but was reluctant to live in a hotel for an extended period of time alone after the surgery.

I inquired about the hospitals in Boston, particularly the Peter Bent Brigham Hospital at Harvard Medical School. My friend, Dr. Tarlov, lived in Boston and offered to let me live at his home after surgery. That was an ideal plan.

I was to have the aortic and mitral valves replaced and bypasses of two obstructed coronary arteries. For this, I decided on the famous heart surgeon, Dr. Lawrence Cohen, a colleague of another friend, a children's heart surgeon at Harvard. In our meeting, Dr. Cohen said, "I'm writing the new chapter on valve replacement for Hodgkin's patients." It was a winning seductive line, which validated my decision to choose him. We selected two artificial, mechanical valves rather than two pig valves to replace the aortic and the mitral valves. That meant I would have to take coumadin, a blood thinner, for the rest of my life to prevent blood from clotting on the artificial valve. Coumadin may cause easy and abundant bleeding, especially nose bleeds. Coumadin also readily causes black and blue marks when the body is struck, even lightly.

I arranged surgery for February 26, 1998 at 7 A.M.

Description of the Heart and Its Four Chambers

The heart, a hollow muscular organ, lies in the center of the chest. The right and the left sides of the heart each have an upper chamber (atrium), which collects blood, and a lower chamber (ventricle), which ejects blood. To ensure that blood flows in only one direction, the ventricles have an inlet and an outlet valve.

The heart's primary functions are to supply oxygen to the body and to rid the body of waste products (carbon dioxide). In short, the heart performs these functions by collecting oxygen-depleted blood from the body and pumping it to the lungs, where it picks up oxygen and drops off carbon dioxide; the heart then collects the oxygen-enriched blood from the lungs and pumps it to the tissues of the entire body.

During each heartbeat, each heart chamber relaxes as it fills, a period called diastole, and then contracts as it pumps blood, a period called systole. The two atria relax together and contract together.

Here's how blood moves through the heart. First, oxygen-depleted, carbon dioxide laden blood from the body flows through the two largest veins (the venae caval) into the right atrium. When this chamber fills, it propels the blood (through the tricuspid valve) into the right ventricle. When the right ventricle fills, it pumps the blood through the pulmonary arteries, which supply the lungs. The blood then flows through tiny capillaries that surround the air sacks in the lungs, absorbing oxygen and giving up carbon dioxide, which is then exhaled. The now oxygen-rich blood flows through the pulmonary veins into the left atrium.

The circuit between the right side of the heart, the lungs and the left atrium is called the pulmonary circulation. When the left atrium fills, it propels the oxygen-rich blood (through the mitral valve) into the left ventricle. When this chamber fills, it pumps the blood through the aortic valve into the aorta, the largest artery in the body. This oxygen-rich blood supplies all of the body except the lungs.

The heart muscle (myocardium) itself receives a fraction of the large volume of blood flowing through the atria and ventricles. A system of arteries and veins (coronary circulation) supplies the myocardium with oxygen-rich blood and then returns oxygen-depleted blood to the right atrium. The right coronary artery and the left coronary artery branch off the aorta to deliver blood (to the myocardium); the cardiac veins empty into the coronary sinus, which returns blood to the right atrium. Because of the great pressure exerted in the heart as it contracts, most blood flow thorough the coronary circulation takes place while the heart is relaxing between beats (during ventricular diastole).[8]

---

[8] Adapted from the *Merck Manual of Medical Information,* 1997, pp. 72–73.

My surgery took ten hours. The operation began with the anesthesiologist, who inserted an arterial line into my wrist to monitor blood pressure and to observe how well my lungs were working. Another line was placed in my neck to measure pressures in the heart and lungs during and immediately after surgery. After I was asleep, the anesthesiologist placed a breathing tube in my windpipe to help breathing during surgery. When I went to sleep, medication was given directly into the lines. The surgery begins at the chest and usually the leg. The chest incision is called a sternotomy. The breastbone (sternum) is sawed through and the ribs are spread. This exposes the heart.

In the operating room, there were also the master surgeon, three surgeon assistants, and a registered nurse. One hour was needed prior to surgery, but the actual operation took about five hours, and the two coronary artery bypasses, or grafts, took additional time. Transporting me to intensive care was another thirty minutes. True or false, it seemed that I awakened mid-surgery to some level of consciousness and could hear the nurse pulling paper towels vigorously and handing them to the surgeon, though I didn't feel any pain. When the surgery was completed, the assistant surgeon informed me that all went well. It was the last time I enjoyed a happy moment.

But disaster struck in the operating room. The heart valves and surrounding tissues responded to high doses of irradiation to treat Hodgkin's Disease with scar formation. Over decades calcium crystals guilt up in the scars. While the old valves were being removed, some crystalline calcium and tissue broke off and traveled through the bloodstream into my head. There, these embolli lodged in small arteries and obstructed the flow of blood. The result was a series of strokes in several or many different parts of the brain. Among other losses I became paralyzed on the left side of my body.

The most frightening part of the post-op experience occurred in intensive care. The cold room kept me awake, and I dreamed there was a corpse lying under the lid of the light blue window seat, where I believed my late mother lay. Another day, I dreamed the room was filled with kelly green liquid and fish swam continuously throughout. Dr. Tarlov loved to fish, and I believed that was the connection with the dream. I suffered many more bad dreams. I needed my family, who lived in Minnesota, but had very few visits from them.

I spent several days in intensive care and was then moved to a regular room where a resident visited to do an evaluation. He wanted to know if I could read words in either regular or large print. I couldn't read either. A neurologist tested me with ten photos asking their identity. I couldn't recognize or differentiate Nixon, Marilyn Monroe, Shirley Temple, nor any other familiar faces. This was the result of the stroke.

I was having a difficult, painful time, so I told the nurse that I was going to commit suicide. I was . . . but how? I learned this is one phrase you cannot use in a hospital. The next day and for several consecutive days, a psychiatrist was asked to visit me. Ultimately, he wondered how I endured all my hardships. I wondered how I did, too. I did not return to my original room, and the patients on that floor thought I had died. I genuinely wished I had. I decided that the hospital was for the chronically ill and could not do anything for me, so an ambulance was called to take me to the Spaulding Rehabilitation Hospital in Boston where I remained as a patient for two months.

Description of a Stroke

When blood flow to the brain is disrupted, brain cells can die or be damaged from lack of oxygen. Brain cells can also be damaged if bleeding occurs in or around the brain. The resulting neurological problems are called cerebrovascular disorders because of the brain (cerebrum) and blood vessel (vascular) involvement.

Insufficient blood supply to parts of the brain for brief periods causes transient ischemic attacks, temporary disturbances in brain function. Because the blood supply is restored quickly, brain tissue doesn't die, as it does in a stroke. A transient ischemic attack is often an early warning sign of a stroke.

In Western countries, strokes are the most common causes of neurologic damage. High blood pressure and atherosclerosis—hardening of the arteries from fatty buildup—are the major risk factors for strokes . . . How a stroke or transient ischemic attack affects the body depends on precisely where in the brain the blood supply was cut off or where bleeding occurred.

A stroke can be either ischemic or hemorrhagic. In an ischemic stroke, the blood supply to part of the brain is cut off because either atherosclerosis or a blood clot has blocked a blood vessel. In a hemorrhagic stroke, a blood vessel bursts, preventing normal flow and allowing blood to leak into an area of the brain and destroy it.[9]

---

[9] *Merck Manual of Medical Information*, 1997, pp. 381-384.

After two months at the rehab center, I accepted the fact that I was disabled. On the left side, I had paresis, which meant I was almost totally paralyzed. My left arm was perpetually stiff and often felt as if bugs were crawling from shoulder to hand. The arm had considerable pain. My left leg was dysfunctional and I could walk only slowly and with assistance.

For five years, I went to pulmonary therapy twice a week, which was the most consistent exercise I had. I swam and attended occupational and physical therapy. I also joined the rheumatoid arthritis swimming class when I visited LaJolla. It was disappointing when I reflected that I used to be a high diver and now I could no longer swim. I organized sessions twice weekly with the occupational and physical therapists, and I took Pilates, believing that in five years I should be well. I wasn't! The five years of exercise did not heal me. The pain did not subside. I still had to walk with a cane and use a wheelchair.

Again, my sisters visited me only once at the hospital in Boston and once at my house in Chicago in a five-year period. I missed them dearly and didn't know the reason they didn't visit.

Physician Two, Dr. Tarlov

Dr. Tarlov is my dear friend and is very attentive. We have known each other for more than twenty years. He discovered me by asking a colleague to introduce him to the outstanding women in Chicago, and Mrs. Whitney Addington, his colleague's wife, introduced him to three women. I was his selection.

Dr. Tarlov is a distinguished internist, but more than that, he was a consistent, loving, and helpful friend. He did everything for me—big and small. We took luxurious vacations and when in Chicago, we attended concerts, plays, and lectures; he also brought me books and flowers. He showed greatness to me at all times. I credit him with my livelihood. Except for Hodgkin's Disease, he helped me with all illnesses—thyroid surgery, breast surgery, open-heart surgery, and stroke.

When I lived at his house after I was released from the hospital, I listened to nature tapes to be soothed. Dr. Tarlov added a small water fountain for relaxation.

Dr. Tarlov has been behind the scenes from 1979 to the present. He helped me with health problems big and small. When I had open heart surgery in 1998 at the Peter Bent Brigham Hospital, Harvard Medical School, and later underwent rehabilitation at the Spaulding Hospital, he visited me daily and brought a special dinner nightly. After discharge from Spaulding Hospital, I lived at his home in Boston while undergoing further rehabilitation treatment. Successful battles against illness are aided substantially by having a good, reliable friend.

Chapter Ten:

Caregivers

It Takes More Than Ten Physicians to Heal a Patient

I needed a good physician, but finding one was a challenge. The two best sources for doctors were references from other doctors and from patients. During twenty years, I had to find more than twenty physicians. The number included three internists for Hodgkin's Disease from Minneapolis and Chicago; five internists between Chicago and Houston; five cardiologists from three different cities; two breast cancer specialists from two Chicago hospitals; three lung specialists from Northwestern Hospital; two physiatrists, one from Chicago and the other from the Spaulding Rehabilitation Hospital in Boston; two thyroid specialists from San Diego and Chicago; a dermatologist; a gynecologist from Chicago; and a dentist from Chicago.

To establish a hierarchy for decision-making and a repository for all new medical files, I chose Dr. James Cohn, an internist, to be the quarterback. Dr. Cohn began his career as an undergraduate at the University of Wisconsin and attended the University of Illinois Medical School. In 1978, he took his internship and residency in internal medicine at Northwestern University. Dr. Cohn taught and was attending physician on an in-patient hospital service for twenty years. His duties included making rounds with students, interns, and residents, and he was responsible for quality care on the service. For a year, he reviewed all new patients to the hospital.

Dr. Cohn's follow-up with patients is exemplary. He never missed a detail, whether it is a return phone call or making an appointment, for which he was always precisely on time. I have great respect for Dr. Cohn's good judgment and common sense. His office is run like a Swiss clock. When you call, his receptionist, Jackie, picks up the phone and provides an answer no matter the subject. Jackie is well informed, pleasant, and helpful. She makes going to the office relaxing. The team gives great service.

A Gracious Caregiver—Henrietta Adarna

At the end of 1998, I arranged to interview a complete stranger, a fifty-year-old Philippine woman, interested in becoming my caregiver. She was unfamiliar to me except that my girlfriend told me about her good work. I made her acquaintance through a brief telephone conversation and a short chat in the living room. The opening transaction was quick. I surprised Rita (Henrietta's nickname) when I said I had no need to interview her further. I was experienced from interviewing many teachers and so was immediately aware that Rita would do a good job since we were compatible people.

Henrietta stood in the dining room in black pants and

a white blouse, and I watched her from where I stood in the living room wearing a short orange skirt and an orange striped blouse. I was trying to complete a book, *The Progressive Legacy*, for publication. I had difficulty typing with only one functional hand. The left hand was paralyzed. Rita had to learn directly from me who I was and what was wrong with me, because there was no one else around to explain the answers to her questions at the time. Her response to me was positive.

Not planning to begin immediately, Rita had arrived without her wardrobe. I wanted her to be the caregiver, so I gave her a light blue nightgown, decorated with four white angels, and a robe. She has stayed with me ever since then—and it's six years later.

In many ways, Rita and I are similar, but we occasionally clash. We are both "responsible perfectionists." But, one morning we laughed until our stomachs hurt. As time passed, we stopped our disputes, but we stopped the laughter, too. Rita often quoted her father's sayings to provide a solution to a problem. For instance, when we were working too hard, she would quote, "Animals with four legs rest more than man with two legs."

Rita serves in many roles. She is the homemaker, ordering groceries and cooking delicious meals. She never serves a meal I dislike. She encourages eight glasses of water a day, many vegetables and fruits. Previously I drank six cups of coffee a day, and now I drink none.

Rita performs the most important task of all—she manages the medication. I take pills four times daily, which Rita arranges in weekly pillboxes. She never makes a mistake ordering, organizing, or dispensing them to me on time. My internist trusts Rita with the prescriptions more

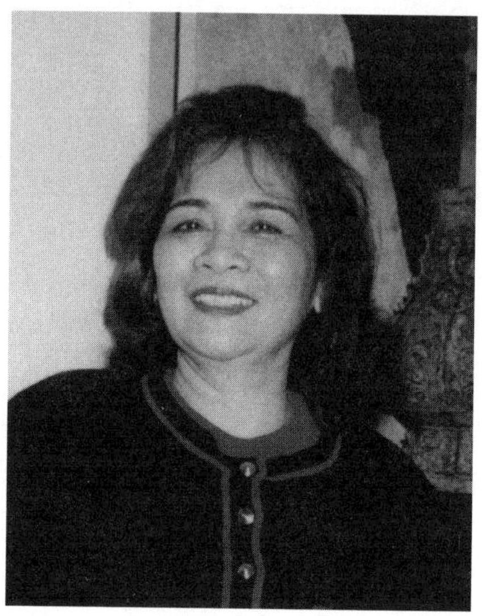

Henrietta I. Adarna, Health Care Provider

than he does me. My physician calls Rita into his office to inform her about new prescriptions, or he phones the changes to her.

Rita also escorts me to the rehabilitation center two or three times weekly for therapy or doctors' appointments. I am on oxygen and can not carry my own canister, so she does. At times, we exercise together at home, and on summer days, we exercise in the heated pool at a friend's house. We walk around the flower garden in the park when we are in Chicago. In late afternoons, we often go out to dinner, to a movie, or to a play.

We also travel together to visit my friends and family. All of them hold her in high esteem and enjoy her company. We travel to LaJolla, Houston, Minneapolis, New York, Dallas, and other destinations. Flying presents certain difficulties, but Rita helps give flying—and my life—a dimension of normalcy, even with the wheelchair and the oxygen, which are required at most times.

Rita is the caregiver par excellence; she takes care of everything in a most gracious way.

Personal Caregiver—Maxine Watson

When at pulmonary therapy, I met a splendid young woman who introduced me to a personal caregiver, Maxine Watson. Maxine began working for me on weekends in early March 2002, and now she works for me every evening and through the night as well.

Maxine's agenda is inclusive. She lotions and dresses me every morning. She does morning chores like fixing the bed and making and serving breakfast. She cleans the bathroom and organizes my makeup before she leaves at 8:00 A.M. Maxine returns at 4:00 P.M. to do evening chores. She is a pro at washing out my clothes, especially my t-shirts and running pants. Often she irons. She gives me my medications in late afternoon and pre-bed. On weekends, Maxine gives me a shower and washes my hair. Maxine is a very capable rehab personal caregiver and a necessary and appreciated person in the household.

Pulmonary Therapy

My physiatrist, Dr. Elliott Roth, recommended pulmonary therapy to improve my breathing following open-heart surgery. Breathing was the most serious problem. Therapy began with a seminar session followed by activities sessions, which included physical exercises on the

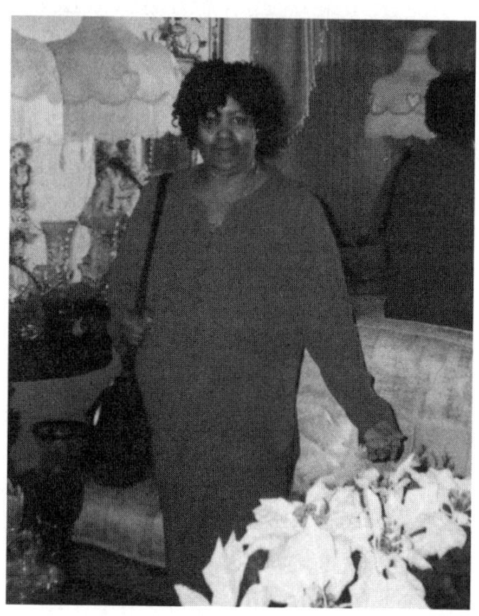

Maxine Watson, Personal Caregiver

bicycle, the treadmill, and with the arm machine. Pulmonary therapy is recommended for at least twelve diseases—Chronic Obstructive Pulmonary Disease (COPD), neurological and neuromuscular diseases, and lung diseases such as cystic fibrosis, bronchitis, asthma, bronchiectasis, emphysema, congestive heart failure, thoracic deformities, post-surgical patients, and lung volume reductive surgery.

The director of the pulmonary clinic at the Chicago Rehabilitation Institute is Enid Silverman and the principal therapist is Brenda Williams. Ms. Williams is a graduate of Malcolm X College and has served the unit for eleven years. Her repertoire is comprehensive. If necessary, she can do a patient assessment, infection control, blood gas analysis, oxygen therapy, airway management, suctioning

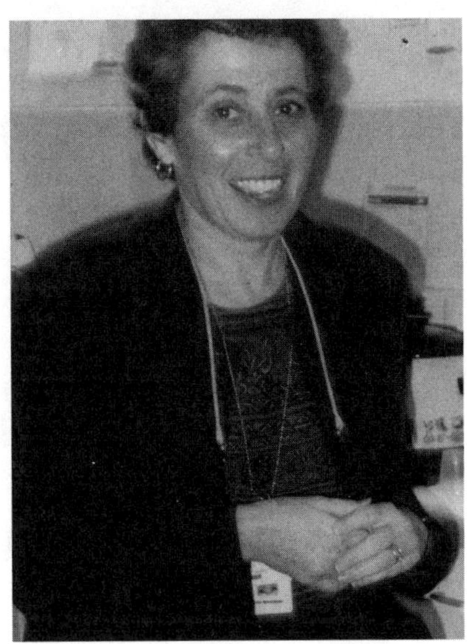

Dr. Enid Silverman, Director

technique, mechanical ventilation, CPR, and pharmacy. She is also the Asthma 101 instructor.

Ms. Williams is a respected therapist and the favorite among the fifty patients served in the program. The schedule consists of twice weekly one-hour sessions, and the course lasts for twelve weeks. Brenda is always busy helping patients or answering the telephone to listen to and advise patients who are unable to attend a session.

She knows her patients well, is attentive to them, and is willing to answer patient questions, which she does knowledgeably and patiently. One member captured her essence in these words, "She wants the patients to feel healthy and encourages them to feel like everyone who is healthy." Brenda is eager to work and often opens the laboratory doors fifteen minutes before the scheduled time so the first session of the day gets an added fifteen minutes.

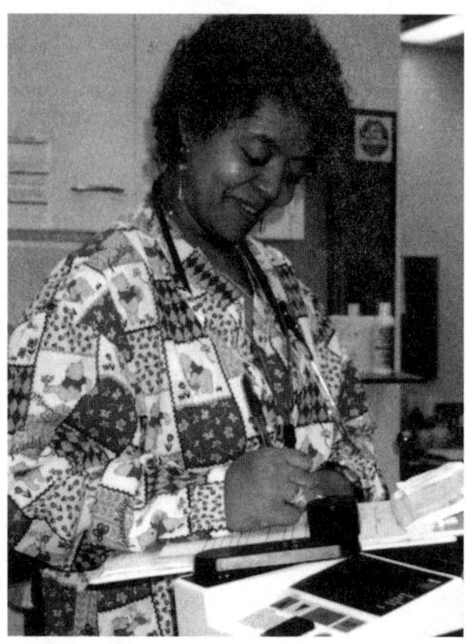

Brenda Williams, Head Nurse

Most patients attend the course regularly. For example, I am attending my sixth year, having missed only a few days.

The pulmonary room is alive. Often, Brenda wears fun shirts decorated with bears, zebras, and other animals. Each month, she posts patients' birthdays, as well as their progress. On the bulletin board, she tacks postcards to show where patients travel to give other patients inspiration. Brenda believes in life and creates a meaningful and a fun hour. She has a positive attitude and a good sense of humor.

Physical Therapy Description

"Unlike pulmonary therapy, physical therapy is carried on in a one-to-one relationship. Physical therapy is a direct form of professional patient care that can be applied in most disciplines of medicine. There are four major objectives to physical therapy: (1) prevention of disability and pain; (2) restoration of function and relief from pain; (3) promotion of healing; and (4) adaptation to permanent disability. Physical therapy is a vital part of the total care for patients with temporary or permanent problems. Physical therapy uses different procedures and modalities beginning with a quantitative evaluation following a stroke, injury, or illness."[10]

At the Chicago Rehabilitation Institute, some twenty patients meet on a one-to-one relationship with a therapist for a forty-five minute session to perform such functions as parallel bars, walking stepways, bouncing balls, and swimming if space permits. Others take Pilates if the PT instructor is qualified. Some use the various exercise machines. I scheduled PT twice weekly or Pilates three times a week when possible. I took PT in a one-hour period for at least three ten-hour sessions. At times, I needed more sessions. Each day, about forty patients awaited appointments.

A turning point in my battle with illness changed the focus from Hodgkin's Disease and radiation therapy, which caused further illnesses, such as breast, thyroid, and skin cancer, to a second emphasis on female problems, with a final concentration on heart and lungs. The first goal in this transition was to change physicians. My first internist in Minneapolis was no longer available, so Dr. James Cohn in Chicago became my internist. My cardiologist in

[10] Physical therapy information by University City Physical Therapy, www.sigafoospt.com.

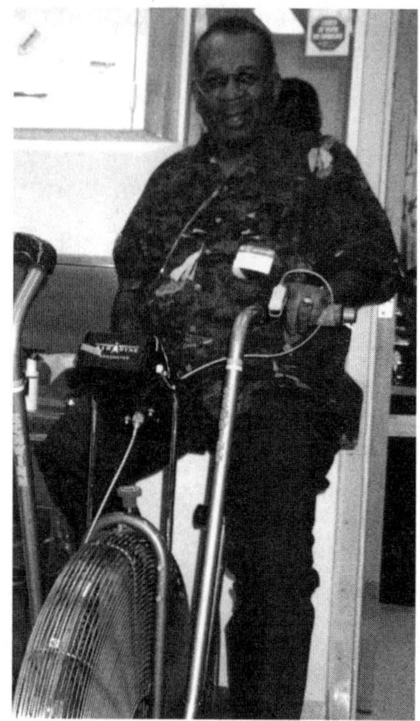

Fred Brown, Patient

Boston, Dr. Patrick O'Gara, was changed to a Chicago cardiologist, Dr. Robert Bonow. I changed my pulmonologist from Dr. Winslow to Dr. Michael Moore, and to the team I added a physiatrist. Dr. Elliott Roth. I was a fortunate person who could select effective physicians for all three situations—Hodgkin's Disease, female problems, and respiratory problems—and choose the best in the city.

After a decade of Hodgkin's Disease, I won the battle. My hair filled in, the red stains on my neck began to fade, and the only scars that remained were those from the breast incision and the thyroid incision.

But a new set of problems intimidated my body. I was ensconced in a handicapped body. The quality of my existence transformed. Now oxygen fed two liters per minute into my lungs consistently. The cord is awkward because of

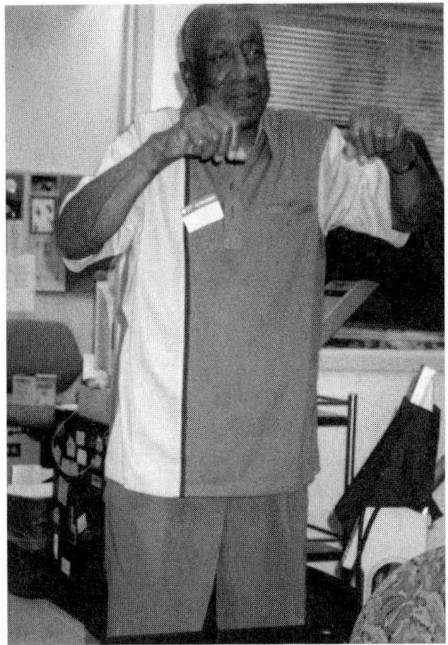

Courtney Tate, Patient

its length, which is several feet long and has to be dragged wherever I walk. I have two large tanks of liquid oxygen delivered to my house every month. When I go to the rehabilitation center twice weekly, we have to take with us a satchel for water, other paraphernalia, and a small canister of oxygen. I have to ride in a wheelchair and require the services of my caretaker everywhere I go. It is difficult to place a wheelchair in the trunk of a cab or a car. In the last two years of illness, I have spent most of my time in a wheelchair. As years four and five post–heart surgery and stroke passed, my body deteriorated more and more, but I could still use the arm machine, the bike, and the treadmill in pulmonary therapy. I was determined to use the treadmill for thirty minutes a session, but in the end, the usage was discontinued because of limitations imposed by my instructor.

To get well, I took pulmonary therapy twice weekly and added three additional sessions to supplement private lessons, which were taken in a group and were comprised of Pilates and balancing exercises to improve walking. I walked through the halls, did exercises on the mat, and tried to walk up and down the stairs. The point was to learn the techniques for personal use at home. At home, I used the chest respiratory vest—a machine that inflates the vest and causes it to thump on my chest rapidly and repetitively to loosen the mucus in my lungs and to aid expectoration.

I also took swimming exercises when they were available. At times, I used the pool at the Rehabilitation Institute, but when it was in use, I swam at the YMCA. My friend built a heated therapeutic pool at his home, where my caretaker helped me swim. I took pulmonary therapy at the Rehabilitation Institute, but physical therapy was taken privately at home. At the end of the fifth year post–heart surgery and stroke, I still continue to struggle with lung and heart disease and the stroke. Few would agree, but the stroke is the worst problem. My left leg is causing mobility problems, but it is my left hand that causes the worst struggle. There is nothing to do about the proverbial pins that run up and down my hand and arm, and I can not alleviate the paralysis that impairs all activity. Some nights I cry in pain. I tried hot wax, a glove, a sponge, clay, and a special vibrating machine. I had to learn to live with pain and with one hand.

Traveling became an additional problem. Oxygen has to be rented from the airlines. The price increased from

$50 to $100 per trip in the five-year period that I have used oxygen. The airlines insist on the use of their oxygen for travel. I can no longer drive a car.

I learned to appreciate medication. My survival depends on it. The worst pill is coumadin. It is necessary, but results in blood marks under the skin after even the slightest bump.

My life changed. I am now handicapped and live in a wheelchair. I can no longer teach. But to fill the empty days, I substitute writing an education history using my one hand only. I have grave difficulty holding manuscript papers with one hand. The papers often flutter to the floor. Finally, I had to hire an editorial assistant to complete *The Progressive Legacy* (2001). Writing and research filled my days for one year, and then the book was published. The book inspired me to establish a school archive (2003), a large collection of documents pertaining to the history of the Frances Parker School since its founding. The school held a book signing to launch the first archives' meeting made up of a group of alumni, teachers, and administrators, who met for a year to fulfill their mission of developing the archives. I provided practically all of the historic documents, which I collected in the process of writing *Between Home and the Community* and *The Progressive Legacy*. Both tasks fulfilled the time meaningfully.

Next, I had to create other tasks. I wrote these memoirs about the battle with illness, which consumed the mornings of 2003 and half of 2004. Using one hand caused me to struggle so I could maintain order and structure, two of my past strengths.

Occupational Therapy Description

"Occupational therapy focuses on the nature, balance, pattern, and context of occupations and activities in the patients' lives. The main aim is to maintain, restore, or create a match beneficial to the individuals between the abilities of the person, the demands of his occupation in the areas of self-care, and the demands of his environment."[11]

Occupational therapy intervention includes thinking about the activity and performing the activity. The visible aspect of the therapy is a series of actions designed to form a recognizable sequence. Ideally, OT is a partnership between the client and the therapist in which both participate actively, increasing the client's responsibility, choice, autonomy, and control over his or her care. OT can include small skill training like tying shoes, folding paper, and the performance and balance of occupations for desired outcome in the areas of self care, productivity, and leisure, that will support recovery, health, well-being and social participation. I scheduled OT twice weekly in a one-to-one relationship. Usually a dozen patients awaited treatment at the Chicago Rehabilitation Institute. I took PT and OT at Schwab, Chicago, and at Hermann Memorial Hospital Southwest, Houston, Texas twice weekly for forty different periods.

Description of Skin Cancer—
Basil Cell Carcinoma (2000)

"Basal cell carcinoma is a cancer that originates

[11] Occupational therapy information by University City Physical Therapy, www.sigafospt.com.

in the lowest layer of the epidermis . . . usually develops on skin surfaces that are exposed to sunlight. The tumors begin as very small, shiny, firm raised growths on the skin (nodules) and enlarge very slowly—sometimes so slowly that they go unnoticed as new growths. However, the growth rate varies greatly from tumor to tumor with some growing as much as one-half-inch in a year. Basal cell carcinomas may ulcerate or form scabs in the center. The borders sometimes take on a pearly white color."[12]

Basal cell carcinoma resulted from radiation treatment. The summer of 2003 was the first time I hid behind long sleeves, long pants, and a large straw hat. I arranged at least three appointments with the dermatologist to burn out the basil cell carcinoma. Because of excessive bleeding due to coumadin, the cancer had to be burned rather than cut. The pain was minimal, but the purple scars would not disappear from my chest.

Illnesses Were a Litany

First one and then another illness occurred—thyroid cancer and breast cancer and skin cancer. Then open-heart surgery and stroke when no teaching could follow, and then pneumonia and further limitations in functioning.

Description of Pneumonia

"Pneumonia is an infection of the lungs that involves the small air sacs (alveoli) and the tissues around them . . . Pneumonia isn't a single illness, but

---

[12] *Merck Manual of Medical Information*, p. 1086.

many different ones, each caused by a different microscopic organism. Usually pneumonia starts after organisms are inhaled into the lungs, but sometimes the infection is carried to the lungs by the bloodstream or it migrates to the lungs directly from a nearby infection . . . Deep breathing exercises and therapy to clear secretions help prevent pneumonia in people at high risk . . ."[13]

One rainy afternoon, after having my hair washed and set, I came home with a chill. I took my temperature, which registered 104 degrees. Rita convinced me that I had to go to the emergency room, where I lay for hours before being admitted to the hospital. Once I was situated in a room, the nurse connected me to several liters of oxygen per minute. Dr. Winslow, my pulmonologist, visited me using a machine to diminish congestion. By mid-afternoon, I was in a state of panic, until Rita wheeled me around the floors to calm me down. I'm unsure of the reason, but I thought I was going to have a nervous breakdown.

When it was time to go home, Rita and I had the wheelchair, oxygen, and too much paraphernalia to carry. When we asked the girl at the desk to help us carry, she snidely commented, "That is the purpose of the family." We didn't have family with us, so we broke the rules and paid a girl to help us carry our things. Two days later, I visited my psychiatrist, whom I had not seen for several months, to discover what disturbed me so much about pneumonia. We were not able to fully determine that.

---

[13] *Merck Manual of Medical Information*, 1997, p. 212.

Chapter Eleven:

A Life Built on the Battleground for Health

The short term consequences of irradiation therapy were benevolent and my Hodgkin's Disease has been cured. However, the long term consequences have been devastating. Every tissue in the path of the irradiation beam continues on a path of deterioration, causing breast, thyroid, and skin cancer in my case, and replacing healthy tissue with non-supple scar tissue in the skin, lung, heart, and everywhere else the beam was directed. The irradiation created the need for heart surgery to replace two valves and bypass two coronary arteries. Slowly but inexorably, my healthy lung tissue has been replaced by scar. Progressively, my capacity to breathe and absorb the oxygen I need for metabolism has dwindled. I now require oxygen by nose cannula twenty-four hours a day. My capacity for exercise is probably five percent of what it had been. In summary, I am either in a wheelchair or in a bed ninety-eight percent of every twenty-four hour period. The battle goes on.

The Battle with Illness

Rarely do friends, family, and intimates develop lasting relationships with a patient. My friends invited me to brunch about once monthly; others invited me to the art institute and out to dinner occasionally. I am less able to accept their invitations now. New friends and colleagues phone from time to time, but the best friends are former students who visit to chat often. In contrast, the mail is more abundant. In juxtaposition, I yearn to be in the presence of my family members more often. Karen telephones every Sunday morning. Linda writes a letter every month.

Inventions

Without my health, my femininity, my breast, my husband, my hair, or a child, I had to reinvent myself for a second time. The first time was the invention of a life before I contracted Hodgkin's Disease. As a youngster, I was already self-made.

I had individualistic tendencies with a bent toward the non-conventional, and a view of the world as if looking into a kaleidoscope. I wanted to do and be everything—a geologist, a scholar, a writer and journalist, a teacher, a dramatist, a dancer, a musician. I tried them all. I was energetic, active, athletic, and in perpetual motion playing tennis once a week and running three times a week, swimming and diving in the summer, ice skating and skiing in the winter, reading, studying, and modern dancing all year, as well as whatever else I could fit into my schedule.

Intellectually, I was also the product of my own making. I chose my own reading lists, insinuated myself into conversations with elder evocative and wise people, engaging with members of all professions to grasp knowledge and opportunities. I attained a master's degree by combining courses at three universities and earned a doctorate at Loyola University where I also taught classes.

Socially, independence and strength were the two strongholds inherited from my family, but I did not want to follow in my mother's footsteps—hers was a life of total sacrifice. The goals my older siblings pursued, working part time at a career and marriage, were not enough for me. My friends' occupations followed the status quo and provided no inspiration. I seriously considered becoming a physician because I held medicine in high regard. Doctors provided good models, but once again, I had to earn my own money for medical school and that would be difficult.

Emotionally, I closed my mind to what I considered ordinary and opened it to opportunity. I listened to my own drumbeats and became my own cheerleader, cheering at times what seemed too difficult to achieve. I never heard, as we now hear mothers tell their children, "You can be whatever you want to be." In fact, the family and I did not discuss goals. I believe my independence emanated from the lack of family involvement. Whether in sickness or in health, my family did not participate in my life.

At the onset of Hodgkin's Disease, I heard the inevitability of my plight, as if listening to a Greek chorus chanting quietly and without interruption a death knoll made up of Browning's poem, about Lazarus' rising from the dead and Job's ultimate challenge, about Edna St. Vincent Millay's, "My Candle Burns at Both Ends," and John Donne's "Death, be not proud," combined with

Hemingway's "It tolls for thee." The chant included some of my own less powerful lines, but the chant did not subside. I got into the habit of referring to myself as "a whitened sepulcher"—beautiful on the outside but rotten on the inside. Habitually, I learned that fear is death's cousin, and self-pity is a debilitating emotion because it is wrapped in the question, "Why me?" The answer bears no fruit, so one might just as well erase the question.

In my extended battle with death, I reflected in retrospect that I was satisfied with the life I had lived—*I never hurt anyone, I helped all I could, and I had a good time traveling throughout the world to line my imagination with silver.*

I developed a knife-cutting discipline and became the possessor of a colossal imagination. I gained strength by fighting illness after illness. Winning one battle strengthened me for the next. Like The Little Engine That Could, my mantra became, "I think I can, I think I can, I can"—and I can.

I was indeed an outlier who lived longer then the ten to twenty-year-old group of survivors. However, irradiated patients are at risk for secondary malignancies like cancer of the breast, basil cell carcinoma, and other diseases. Because radiation injures normal tissue, it can give rise to cancers and serious heart and lung problems.

By the time I reached age forty, health problems compounded; each illness created another health issue. At age twenty, Hodgkin's Disease resulted in the loss of physical health and destruction caused by radiation. It also resulted in the loss of the first love of my life. At age thirty, Hodgkin's Disease, cervical cancer, and endometriosis culminated in a hysterectomy, which resulted in the forfeiture of my husband. By my mid-forties, radiation for Hodgkin's Disease resulted in thyroid and breast cancers.

Intermittently for twenty years, I was living on determination, unwilling to give up. More importantly, I was thriving on teaching students of all ages. Teaching immigrants at Alexander Ramsey High School helped these students learn to adapt to their environment and to eventually soar. Teaching girls at the girls' school helped them to broaden their horizons. Educating students at private school taught them to combine new and old ideas in an interdisciplinary manner. In college teaching, the curriculum was essentially based on texts to be closely followed. In all four venues, the students grew and I grew. The same way that Lance Armstrong made the bike his central focus, I made teaching my central focus.

Lessons Learned through Illness

Illness taught usual and unusual health lessons. One lesson was to behave like a healthy individual. Patients have a tendency to talk about illness, and people have the tendency to dislike and avoid individuals with illnesses, so it's important not to talk about sickness frequently and randomly. People are disinterested in patients' problems. Therefore, find other topics to engage people as if a healthy person.

Another lesson I drew from my past was discipline—discipline in all brands of life—establishing a schedule; rising on time; eating three well balanced meals daily; balancing work, play, and study; never missing a doctor's appointment; and other regularities of life that might have been treated haphazardly before, but not now. Discipline was my strongest habit, but it was difficult to alter my behavior from what I wanted to schedule to what I should schedule. I was juggling six physicians and five therapists, but the best guide and greatest support sustaining me through my battles was fantasy. Like a diorama, I visualized a dream and tried to fill in the spaces. I fantasized that I would be healthy in five years and believed it. Now I am in the middle of the sixth year and regret that I no longer am capable of teaching after five years. I worry that I am going down hill physically.

According to Dr. Kubler Ross, the Swiss philosopher (and recently deceased) and an authority on death and dying, there are five stages—grief, denial, anger, bargaining, depression, and acceptance. I transpired through all stages. As the years passed, I was challenged by more illnesses.

The fantasy was fragmented from ages twenty through age sixty-five. Illness shaped and re-shaped my body and my dream.

This litany of illnesses was textbook, and I named Hodgkin's Disease "the mother of all cancers." The profession had not identified Hodgkin's Disease as a cancer in the usual sense of the word. Throughout the next four decades, three more cancers transformed me into a different kind of person—physically, emotionally, intellectually, and spiritually.

Chapter 12:

It Takes More Than Ten Physicians to Heal a Patient

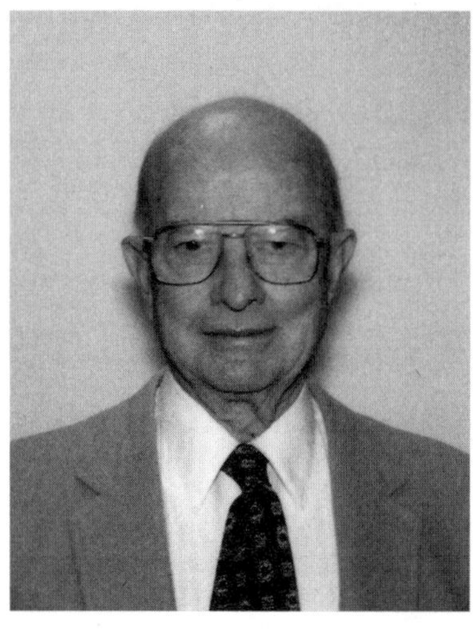

G. Donn Mosser, MD
Radiation Therapist

He was not the first physician I ever saw, but he was the major force in my medical care from the start of my illnesses. His radio-therapeutic wizardry cured my Hodgkin's disease before it was known **that could be done**. He remains in my thoughts practically every day as a revered physician and humanitarian.

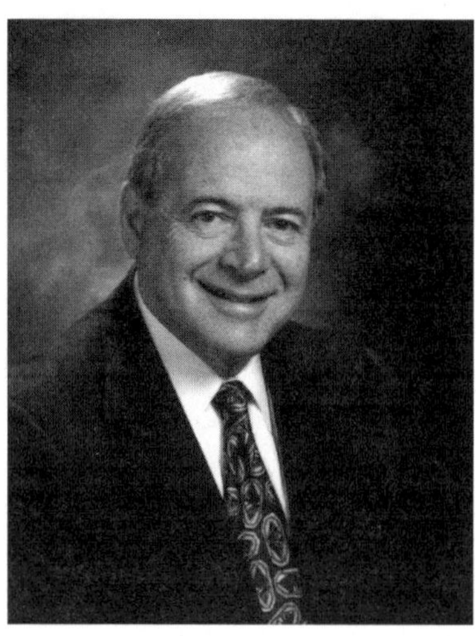

Alvin R. Tarlov, MD
Internist

Great friend in good times, savior in bad, valued companion always.

Edwin Kaplan, MD
Endocrine Surgeon

He is a superb thyroid surgeon and a warm and personal physician. He cured my thyroid cancer while preserving my parathyroid glands, no small accomplishment.

Wilson Hartz, MD
Surgeon

A fine, careful, and effective surgeon, excellent communicator, compassionate physician, he cured my breast cancer and conquered my angry gall bladder.

Nancy L. Furey, MD
Dermatologist

Common sense, good judgment and master of all the tools of her trade, she has tamed my skin cancers.

Patrick O'Gara, MD
Cardiologist

Cardiologist extraordinaire, his mastery of the high art of clinical cardiology has earned the respect of the cardiac fraternity nationwide. He provided oversight for every step of my cardiac care in Boston.

Lawrence Cohen, MD
Cardiac Surgeon

Cardiac surgeon of recognized eminence, he removed two of my radiation weary, encrusted, stone-hard heart valves using orthopedic shears and sewed in their place two manmade replacements. They have been thumping regularly and audibly for six years and keep my circulation going in the intended direction. The price? A stroke during the surgery.

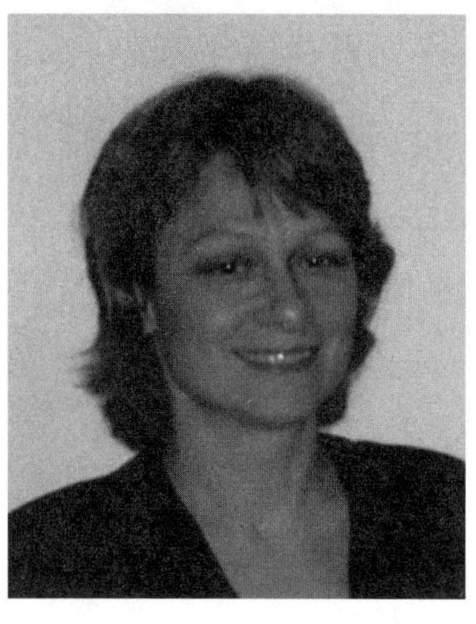

Donna Barber, MD, DDS
Dentist

Irradiation therapy several decades ago sprayed some rays upward into my jaw which has weakened my teeth. She repairs cracks, prevents bad things from happening, and encourages me.

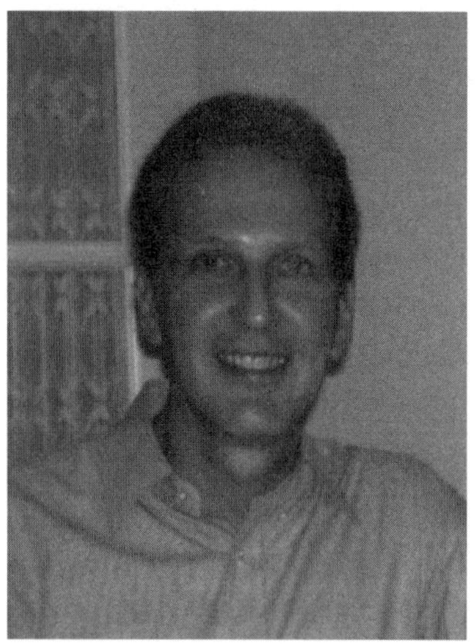

James H. Cohn, MD
Internist

A fine internist, he is the captain of my team. He makes the decisions on when and which consultant to see, what medical step to take, and which medicines to add, subtract, or change dosage. His skills as a physician set a high standard in his office which his office staff has adapted as their own. It is tremendously reassuring and therapeutic just to visit him and the office.

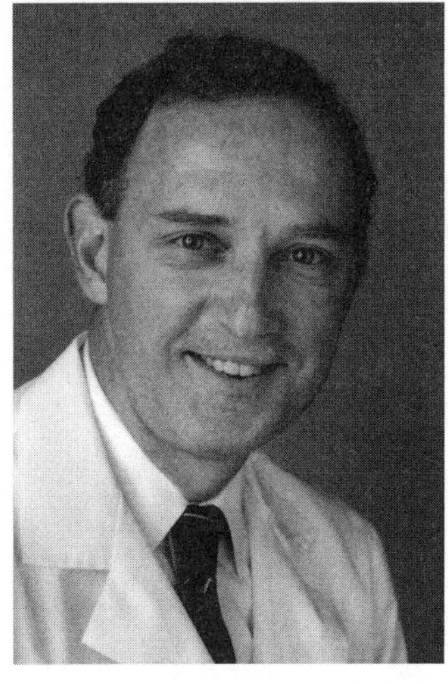

Robert O. Bonow, MD
Cardiologist

He exudes high standards and understandable professional stature. Within the cardiology mob he is part of the O'Garista family operating out of the American College of Cardiology in two major medical cities, Boston and Chicago. He fine-tunes my cardiovascular system and the hydrodynamics associated with it.

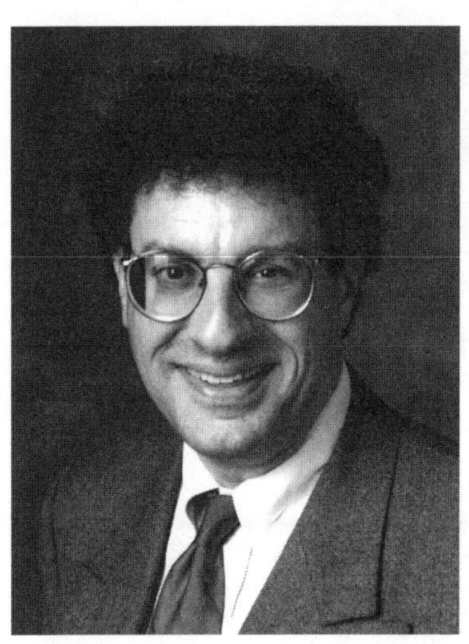

Elliot Roth, MD
Physiatrist

He is an extraordinarily fine person. Physiatrists rehabilitate. We have tried everything and continue to search for new things, or old, that will help. I have a special warm spot in my heart for him because he never gives up.

Christopher Winslow, MD
Pulmonary Physician

He has strong analytic and diagnostic skills that help manage lung problems. He cured my acute pneumonia which I thought was going to take my life.

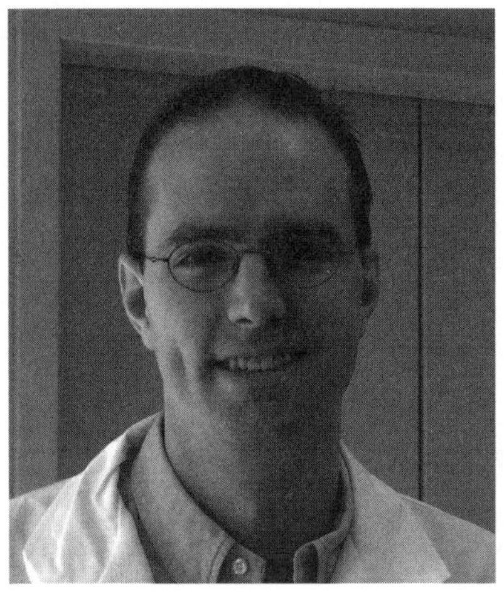

Michael Moore, MD
Pulmonologist

He is the newest physician in my repertoire. He applies his medical skills seriously. He will be challenged by my medical condition, but I think he can succeed.